Cancer Research and Clinical Trials in Developing Countries

Daniela Cristina Stefan

Editor

Cancer Research and Clinical Trials in Developing Countries

A Practical Guide

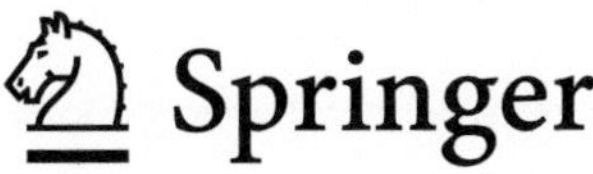 Springer

Editor
Daniela Cristina Stefan, MD, PhD
South African Medical Research Council, Francie van Zyl
Parrow, Cape Town, South Africa

ISBN 978-3-319-18442-5   ISBN 978-3-319-18443-2   (eBook)
DOI 10.1007/978-3-319-18443-2

Library of Congress Control Number: 2015956613

Springer Cham Heidelberg New York Dordrecht London
© Springer International Publishing Switzerland 2016
This work is subject to copyright. All rights are reserved by the Publisher, whether the whole or part of
the material is concerned, specifically the rights of translation, reprinting, reuse of illustrations, recitation,
broadcasting, reproduction on microfilms or in any other physical way, and transmission or information
storage and retrieval, electronic adaptation, computer software, or by similar or dissimilar methodology
now known or hereafter developed.
The use of general descriptive names, registered names, trademarks, service marks, etc. in this publication
does not imply, even in the absence of a specific statement, that such names are exempt from the relevant
protective laws and regulations and therefore free for general use.
The publisher, the authors and the editors are safe to assume that the advice and information in this book
are believed to be true and accurate at the date of publication. Neither the publisher nor the authors or the
editors give a warranty, express or implied, with respect to the material contained herein or for any errors
or omissions that may have been made.

Printed on acid-free paper

Springer International Publishing AG Switzerland is part of Springer Science+Business Media
(www.springer.com)

Dedicated to the millions who are in need of better health care through the progress of science.

Contents

Contributors

Rajendra A. Badwe, M.S. Department of Surgical Oncology, Tata Memorial Centre, Parel, Mumbai, Maharashtra, India

Ioana Berindan-Neagoe, Ph.D. Research Center for Functional Genomics and Translational Medicine, Iuliu Hatieganu University of Medicine and Pharmacy, Cluj Napoca, Cluj, Romania

Matthys Botha Unit for Gynaecological Oncology, Department of Obstetrics and Gynecology, Tygerberg Hospital and University of Stellenbosch, Cape Town, South Africa

Cornelia Braicu Research Center for Functional Genomics, Biomedicine and Translational Medicine, "Iuliu Hatieganu" University of Medicine and Pharmacy, Victor Babes, Cluj-Napoca, Romania

Ahmed Elzawawy, M.D. Ph.D. Med Department of Clinical Oncology and Nuclear Medicine, Faculty of Medicine, Suez Canal University, Ismailia and Alsoliman Clinical and Radiation Oncology Centre, Port Said, Egypt

Wei Han, Ph.D. Department of Epidemiology and Statistics, Institute of Basic Medical Sciences, Chinese Academy of Medical Sciences and School of Basic Medicine, Peking Union Medical College, Beijing, China

Jingmei Jiang, Ph.D. Department of Epidemiology and Statistics, Institute of Basic Medical Sciences, Chinese Academy of Medical Sciences and School of Basic Medicine, Peking Union Medical College, Beijing, China

Rebecca Johnson, B.Sc., M.B.Ch.B., Ph.D. Oxford University Hospitals NHS Trust, John Radcliffe Hospital, Oxford, Oxfordshire, UK

David Kerr, M.D., D.Sc., F.R.C.P., F.Med.Sci. Radcliffe Department of Medicine, University of Oxford, John Radcliffe Hospital, Oxford, Oxfordshire, UK

Gilberto Lopes, M.D., M.B.A. Oncoclinicas do Brasil, São Paulo, SP, Brazil

Mala Ali Mapatano, M.D., M.P.H., Ph.D. Kinshasa School of Public Health, Department of Nutrition, Kinshasa, Democratic Republic of Congo

Zandile June-Rose Mchiza, Ph.D. Med. Population Health, Health Systems and Innovation, Human Sciences Research Council of South Africa, Cape Town, South Africa

Fedor Moissenko, M.D., Ph.D. Laboratory of Nanobiotechnology, St. Petersburg Academic University—Nanotechnology Research and Education Center of the Russian Academy of Sciences, St. Petersburg, NA, Russia

Patricia Moretto, M.D., M.Sc. Oncology, Caxias do Sul University Foundation, Caxias do Sul General Hospital, Caxias do Sul, RS, Brazil

Jean Marie Kabongo Mpolesha, M.D., Ph.D. Department of Pathology, University Hospital, Mbanza-Lemba, Kinshasa, Democratic Republic of Congo

Philip C. Nasca, Ph.D. School of Public Health, State University of New York, USA

Gouri Pantvaidya, M.S., M.R.C.S. Department of Surgical Oncology, Tata Memorial Centre, Parel, Mumbai, Maharashtra, India

C.S. Pramesh, M.S., F.R.C.S. Department of Surgical Oncology, Tata Memorial Centre, Parel, Mumbai, Maharashtra, India

Priya Ranganathan, M.D. Department of Anaesthesiology, Critical Care and Pain, Tata Memorial Centre, Parel, Mumbai, Maharashtra, India

Luis A. Salicrup, M.S., Ph.D. Center for Global Health, National Cancer Institute, National Institutes of Health, Rockville, MD, USA

Eduardo Seleiro, Ph.D. International Agency for Research on Cancer, Lyon, France

Daniela Cristina Stefan, M.D., Ph.D. South African Medical Research Council, Francie van Zyl, Parrow, Cape Town, South Africa

Ciprian Tomuleasa, M.D., Ph.D. Research Center for Functional Genomics and Translational Medicine, Iuliu Hatieganu University of Medicine and Pharmacy, Cluj Napoca, Cluj, Romania

John J. Welch, M.D., Ph.D. Center for Global Health, National Cancer Institute, National Institutes of Health, Rockville, MD, USA

Gustavo Werutsky, M.D. Latin American Cooperative Oncology Group, Porto Alegre, RS, Brazil

Fang Xue, Ph.D. Department of Epidemiology and Statistics, Institute of Basic Medical Sciences, Chinese Academy of Medical Sciences and School of Basic Medicine, Peking Union Medical College, Beijing, China

Michèle Desire Zeier, M.B., Ch.B., Ph.D. Department of Obstetrics and Gynecology, Faculty of Health Sciences, University of Stellenbosch, Cape Town, South Africa

Biao Zhang, M.S. Department of Epidemiology and Statistics, Institute of Basic Medical Sciences, Chinese Academy of Medical Sciences and School of Basic Medicine, Peking Union Medical College, Beijing, China

Chapter 1
Introduction: The Need to Conduct Cancer Research in Developing Countries

Daniela Cristina Stefan

Most cancers appear in the low- and middle-income countries, simply because of the seven billion inhabitants of our planet, almost six billion fall within that income category. The International Agency for Research on Cancer (IARC) estimated that, out of the 14.1 million new cancer cases which occurred in 2012 internationally, 57 % (eight million) occurred in less-developed regions as well as 65 % of cancer deaths [1]. When incidence and mortality percentages are considered together, it seems clear that the death rates among people with cancer are comparatively higher in developing than in more developed countries.

The estimations for the future are not optimistic. IARC predicts that by 2025, the annual number of new cancers will increase to 19.3 million, and the developing countries' share will be even larger [2]. This will be mainly due to increasing life expectancy in those populations, associated with urbanization and increased adoption of unhealthy lifestyles. The considerable economic cost of lost years due to disability and death will detract from the prospects of development in low- and middle-income countries.

A slow awakening to the reality of cancer becoming a prominent health danger is evident in these countries. Cancer registration and national cancer control plans are materializing progressively and new cancer centers are opening. But the hurdles to overcome remain high: mass awareness needs to be created and preventative measures need to be instituted while infrastructure, equipment, medicines, and skills are far from adequate to respond to treatment needs. And this is all taking place in an environment where financial constraints are prevalent.

Often, in a low- or middle-income setting and in a markedly different culture, modalities of screening, diagnosis and treatment of cancers, imported from resource-rich countries, are not working. Even in those rich countries, it is now obvious that

D.C. Stefan, M.D., Ph.D. (✉)
South African Medical Research Council, Francie van Zyl,
Parrow, Cape Town, South Africa
e-mail: Cristina.Stefan@mrc.ac.za

© Springer International Publishing Switzerland 2016
D.C. Stefan (ed.), *Cancer Research and Clinical Trials in Developing Countries*, DOI 10.1007/978-3-319-18443-2_1

the cost of some therapies is beyond the reach of many. It is urgent that we find innovative solutions for the specific challenges of tackling the cancer burden in limited resource environments.

Additionally, the incidence of various cancers is substantially different in the less-developed populations. In limited-resource environments, infection-related cancers are more prevalent. While in resource-rich populations these types of cancer constitute around 10 % of the total burden of malignant disease, in other parts of the world they make up 25 % of the total number of new cancers. Human papilloma virus, known to be associated with cancer of the uterine cervix, the hepatitis B virus, which is implicated in the pathogenesis of hepatocellular carcinoma, Epstein-Barr virus, connected with Burkitt lymphoma, and human herpes virus 8 which is responsible for Kaposi sarcoma—to mention just some infectious agents—are more prevalent in developing countries. The prevalence of many of these is also increased by the HIV/AIDS epidemic. Numerous other cancers are unequally distributed around the globe.

Answers to the specific issues of cancer control in developing countries can only be found by means of sustained research, carried out by local teams, who have a detailed knowledge of the people, their language, and their mores, as well as knowledge of the epidemiology of cancer and of the specifics of the local cancer health-care system. However, the capacity for such research still has to be developed in many cases.

Many developing countries have established relationships with resource-rich nations in the quest to conduct collaborative research addressing major health issues. Such common activities, generically known as "North–south partnerships," offer the advantage of better access to grants and of assisting with developing research infrastructure and cadres in the southern country. Numerous examples of perennial, successful collaborations exist. However, the experience of such partnerships has shown that the objective of developing research capacity in the low-resource partner is not always attained, the largest share of the grants being used for processing samples in northern laboratories or for salaries of northern scientists who were dispatched to either collect samples or direct the research in the southern country [3]. Moreover, research questions are often formulated to suit the needs of the northern donor country rather than those of the southern partner.

Acknowledging the need to support local scientists, many developing countries adhered, in 2008, to the Bamako Call to Action on Research for Health. Governments pledged at least 2 % of their health budgets for research, while donors agreed to earmark 5 % of their donations for the same purpose and all signatories promised to strengthen their capacity for research [4]. Such initiatives showed encouraging results: for example, scientometric analysis of African research indicates that from 1996 to 2012, the yearly number of published scientific papers listing at least one African author has more than quadrupled [5]. At the same time, however, Africa's share in the global scientific output reached just 2.3 % [5].

Such results cannot be confidently used to characterize cancer research. There is still a long road ahead, and this book hopes to contribute one step. Designed to suit the needs of new researchers in developing countries, the content covers the essentials of conducting research in diverse cultural, regulatory, and financial circumstances. In order to have access to firsthand experience, contributions were solicited from scientists who have worked in or are presently working in low- and middle-income countries. More specifically, we attempted to collate contributions from Brazil, Russia, India, China, and South Africa. These, the so-called BRICS countries, while possessing a research capacity superior to other developing nations, can share their valuable recent experience of overcoming the particular challenges encountered in such environments.

References

1. IARC. Globocan 2012. Cancer fact sheets. All cancers (excluding non-melanoma skin cancer). Estimated incidence, mortality and prevalence worldwide in 2012. 2012. globocan.iarc.fr/Pages/fact_sheets_cancer.aspx. Accessed 1 May 2015.
2. IARC. Latest world cancer statistics (IARC Press release No. 223). Global cancer burden rises to 14.1 million new cases in 2012: marked increase in breast cancer must be addressed. 12 Dec 2013. http://www.iarc.fr/en/media-centre/pr/2013/pdfs/pr223_E.pdf?utm_source=dlvr.it&utm_medium=tumblr. Accessed 5 Feb 2015.
3. Stefan DC, Trimble T. Developing and maintaining effective North–south, South-South and South-South–north partnerships. In: Rebbeck TR, editor. Handbook for cancer research in Africa. Brazzaville: WHO Regional Office for Africa, AORTIC; 2013.
4. The Global Ministerial Forum on Research for Health: the Bamako call to action on research for health. Bamako, Mali, 17–19 Nov 2008. http://www.who.int/rpc/news/BAMAKOCALLTOACTIONFinalNov24.pdf. Accessed 1 May 2015.
5. Schemm Y. Africa doubles research output over past decade, moves towards a knowledge-based economy. Research Trends. 2013;35. http://www.researchtrends.com/issue-35-december-2013/africa-doubles-research-output/. Accessed 6 Feb 2015.

Chapter 2
Steps of a Research Study: From Research Question to Publication

Priya Ranganathan, Gouri Pantvaidya, C.S. Pramesh, and Rajendra A. Badwe

Abstract The steps of a research study include a number of elements which are described starting from generating a research idea to final publication. The journey of good clinical research goes through a systematic circle of generating a research idea and framing a research question, thorough literature review, designing the study, writing the research protocol and getting ethics approval, the actual conduct of the study, monitoring, study completion, data analysis, and finally, publication of the results. This chapter takes the reader through each of these components briefly and gives a broad overview of the entire research process.

Keywords Steps of a research study • Research question • Design of the study • Writing a research protocol • Conduct of the study • Monitoring • Study completion • Data analysis • Publication

Introduction

Biomedical research, like any other area of research in science and technology, is crucial for progress in medicine. However, there are three important reasons why biomedical clinical research is completely distinct from any other field of scientific research. First, given the variability between human beings, much of clinical research necessarily needs to be done using human beings as subjects, making it extremely challenging, and bringing a unique set of logistic and ethical complexities. Second, biological uncertainty is so much broader and deeper than in, say,

P. Ranganathan, M.D. (✉)
Department of Anaesthesiology, Critical Care and Pain, Tata Memorial Centre,
Dr. Ernest Borges Road, Parel, Mumbai, Maharashtra 400012, India
e-mail: RANGANATHANP@TMC.GOV.IN

G. Pantvaidya, M.S., M.R.C.S. • C.S. Pramesh, M.S., F.R.C.S. • R.A. Badwe, M.S.
Department of Surgical Oncology, Tata Memorial Centre,
Dr. Ernest Borges Road, Parel, Mumbai, Maharashtra 400012, India
e-mail: docgouri@gmail.com; prameshcs@tmc.gov.in; badwera@tmc.gov.in

© Springer International Publishing Switzerland 2016
D.C. Stefan (ed.), *Cancer Research and Clinical Trials in Developing Countries*, DOI 10.1007/978-3-319-18443-2_2

physics, engineering, or computing that logic and technological progress does not always imply true scientific progress—these still needs to be tested formally in a clinical setting. Finally, the results of clinical research have such far-reaching impact on human lives that factors beyond mere numbers come into play while determining the "success" or "failure" of a human clinical research experiment.

Generating and Framing a Research Idea

The first, and probably the most exciting step in the process of biomedical research, is to generate a research idea. Elementary as this may sound, it is not always easy to come up with thoughts that are truly innovative and path-breaking. Clinical research ideas primarily originate from two sources: first, routine patient care brings forth unmet needs in clinical practice—specific problems faced by clinicians in diagnostics and therapeutics, and careful analysis of unexpected clinical observations can be the stimulus for some genuinely important research ideas; second, from previous research either in the same or an allied field—most clinical research involves carrying forward the results of previous work on the subject. Good research questions often occur in the most unlikely of situations—in the midst of a busy outpatient clinic, over breakfast with a colleague, while on a long, boring flight, etc.; however, some of the best ideas occur during formal or informal discussions with peers and fellow clinicians/researchers. What is important is to have an open mind, receptive to new thoughts and ideas. A good clinical researcher needs to be inquisitive and skeptical—inquisitive enough to want to know the whys, hows, and why nots; and skeptical enough to question existing beliefs and challenge dogma.

Characteristics of a Good Research Question

The characteristics of a good research idea are that it should ideally fulfill the "FINER" criteria. "FINER" is an acronym standing for Feasible, Interesting, Novel, Ethical, and Relevant. Feasibility involves issues like whether adequate numbers of patients are likely to be recruited, whether the research team has adequate expertise to design and conduct the study, whether it is affordable in terms of time and money, and whether the project is manageable in scope [1]. The research question also needs to be interesting not only to the principal investigator, but also to the research team as a whole (to maintain motivation throughout the study) and to the clinical community at large (to make the effort worthwhile). Novelty of a research idea is probably the most difficult criterion to fulfill, and while a completely innovative approach is the dream of any researcher, studies which confirm or refute the findings of other studies or extend previous findings are meaningful contributions. That the research needs to be ethical sounds elementary, but this is often not as black and white as it seems. Research ethics are an extremely controversial topic and what is ethical in one culture may not be so in another. Finally, the research question needs to be relevant to advancing scientific knowledge on the topic, future research directions, and clinical and health policy in general [1].

Framing a Research Question

Framing the research question is an integral part of the process of refining a research idea, but is not always easy. A good research question can help a researcher to select the appropriate study design and statistical analysis, thereby permitting him/her to answer the fundamental research question unambiguously. Research questions frequently originate from unmet needs either in routine clinical care or in research. This is a useful exercise which forces the researcher into thinking about the research idea and putting it in the form of a "research question," which can be answered by an appropriate study design. It also enables a vague research idea to be crystallized into a specific and focused research question based on a sound hypothesis. The research "hypothesis" and the research "question" are intricately linked. The research hypothesis is the answer or the result expected from the study—this is only a hunch, and the results may or may not actually confirm the hunch, but the process is expected to answer the question one way or another.

Constituents of a Good Research Question

A good research question needs to be structured and the PICOT approach gives a formal framework. The constituents of PICOT include Population, Intervention, Comparator, Outcomes, and Timeframe. This approach helps make the process of framing a research question concise and systematic and ensures that all the components of a research question are addressed [2]. Framing the research question itself clarifies the thought process behind the research idea systematically and methodically [3, 4].

Population

One of the first steps in formulating a research question is to identify the population where the researcher intends to conduct the study. Will all patients with a disease condition or a more select subset be the potential study subjects? Defining the population is effectively identifying the major eligibility criteria for the study. It is important to strike a balance between having eligibility criteria that make the population as similar to each other as possible (homogeneity) and enabling the results of the study to be generalizable to most patients with the disease condition.

Intervention

What is the (new) intervention that is the subject of the research study? Clearly defining the exact intervention is important for further development of the research idea, for the design of the study, and for future replication of the study by other researchers.

Comparator

What is the reference treatment to which the new treatment will be compared? Will it be the existing standard of care? Will it be to placebo in a condition where no effective (or acceptable) treatment currently exists?

Outcomes

Defining the outcomes at the beginning of a study is crucial—and is different for different study designs. While for a phase III cancer trial, the outcome of interest may be overall survival, it could well be dose finding for a phase I study and toxicity for a phase II study. A good primary outcome should be valid, reliably measureable, specific, reproducible and, most importantly, appropriate to the research question.

Timeframe

Defining the timeframe involves both the timeframe for data collection and by extension, that of the outcome measures. The timeframe needs to be long enough to measure relevant outcomes. Not all research questions have the "T" of PICOT, and therefore have the PICO format.

The advantage of using the PICOT framework is that it converts a vague research idea into something more focused (and answerable) and gives a definite structure to the research question. To give an example, the research idea might be "Chemotherapy could be useful in early lung cancer." Thinking systematically about this idea and about possible ways to reach the truth forces the researcher to think of more specific issues: which patients are we planning to study?; will it include non-small cell or small cell lung cancer?; will all patients with early lung cancer be included or should the study be restricted to those patients who have undergone complete surgical resection?; should the chemotherapy be given prior to or after surgery?; how many cycles of chemotherapy should be given?; what kind of chemotherapy should be administered?, etc. The researcher is then forced to state his idea as a research question with a formal hypothesis. The hypothesis might be that the addition of adjuvant chemotherapy improves 5-year survival in patients undergoing surgery for stage I, II, IIIA non-small cell lung cancer (NSCLC). The research question is then specified as "Will three cycles of postoperative platinum-based doublet chemotherapy improve 5-year survival compared to surgery alone in patients who have undergone complete surgical resection for stage IB to IIB NSCLC?"—clearly a much more defined idea than "Will chemotherapy be useful in early lung cancer?"

A useful template of PICOT for an interventional study would therefore be: *"In _____(P), how does ______(I) compared with ______(C) affect ______ (O) over ____ (T) period of time?"* [5].

In the example above, the PICOT constituents are as follows

Population: Patients who have undergone complete surgical resection for stage IB to IIB non-small cell lung cancer.

Intervention: Three cycles of postoperative platinum-based doublet chemotherapy.

Comparator: Patients treated with surgery alone.

Outcomes: Overall survival.

Timeframe: 5-year survival.

While the actual question may vary depending on the research idea, the PICOT framework provides a useful skeleton for the entire research study.

Literature Search

The next step after defining the research question is to perform a thorough literature search on the topic of interest. A "literature search" is a process of searching for existing information and evidence related to the research question.

Need for Performing a Literature Search

A literature search will help to:

- Find earlier published research done on the same or similar topics: this is the most important reason for a thorough literature search. If the research idea has already been adequately addressed, repeating the same study would be a waste of resources, both time and money. Also a critical appraisal of the literature will contribute to the better understanding of the research area and not just accepting blindly the results. Find lacunae in available research thereby helping to modify the research question: contrary to the point above, if previous research on the same idea has been performed with several methodological errors, it justifies repeating the research without the flaws of previous studies, provided the question is worth answering.
- Highlight controversies in the existing literature.
- Help design investigations, treatment protocols, questionnaires, and end points for the research question.

Process of a Literature Search

The process of a literature search involves the following steps:

Step 1: Defining the Right Research Question

The importance of this step cannot be overemphasized. As described, identifying the right research question is the key to a focused literature search. The absence of a well-defined question will provide a literature search that is muddled and confusing. For example, a nursing team would like to conduct a research study on surgical site infections. If the research question is not adequately defined to include the PICOT criteria, the literature search will give information on surgical site infections in all procedures from mastoidectomy to varicose veins surgery. This would become unwieldy. Sifting out the necessary from the unnecessary would then become strenuous, time-consuming, and a deterrent to carrying out the next steps of the search.

Step 2: Planning the Literature Search

Prior to starting the search, the approach to the search should be defined. There are different methods to perform the literature search like a systematic search, where all relevant material is looked for, or a targeted search, which is very selective and focused. One would generally use a combination of the two approaches.

Step 3: Using the Available Research Tools Appropriately

This is probably the most important step of the literature search. There are a wide variety of search engines available on the internet. It is important to be able to use the right keywords and the appropriate search engine for a usable result.

Keywords—These are two or three key terms, which describe the topic for the search. These do not necessarily have to be single words; they could be a combination of two or three words or a phrase.

For example, while searching for literature on "Screening tools for breast cancer in the United States," the keywords could possibly be—breast cancer/screening/United States. These keywords may need to be refined depending on the results, to include more specific terms. In the above example, one may need to include terms like mammography, breast MRI, etc. While choosing keywords, synonyms and similar sounding terms may be used to refine the search.

Boolean Logic [6]

When searching for literature in a database, Boolean logic refers to the logical relationship between search terms. The Boolean operators are AND, OR, NOT. These have to be typed in upper case to connect the keywords or search terms. Multiple Boolean operators can be used in one search term. "AND" is used to find research articles where all the keywords are used. In the above example, if one is looking for research articles evaluating the role of mammography and breast MRI for screening, the search term would be "mammography AND breast MRI AND screening." "OR" is used to find research articles which have at least one of the keywords used. In the above example, when searching for tools for screening, one could use "mammography OR breast MRI" and citations on either mammography or breast MRI will be displayed. "NOT" is used when the keyword after the NOT needs to be eliminated. In the above example, if the topic of interest is the role of mammography in breast cancer screening and not in diagnosing it, the search term would be "mammography AND screening NOT diagnostics."

Developing and Writing a Protocol

Definition

A research protocol is defined as "a document that describes the objective(s), design, methodology, statistical considerations, and organization of a trial" [7]. It is the single most important document in clinical research. The study protocol helps readers to understand why the study needs to be done and how it will be carried out.

Why Is a Research Protocol Needed? [8, 9]

A research protocol is needed for the following reasons:

- It outlines the scientific rationale and objectives of the study.
- It standardizes the research methodology and ensures consistency during the study.
- It ensures that investigators think about and plan all aspects of the study.
- It is necessary for ethics committee approval.
- It is essential for funding applications.
- It helps in writing the manuscript.

While industry-sponsored studies generally have ready protocols with minimum input from investigators, it is the responsibility of the investigator to write the protocol for investigator-initiated studies.

Elements of the Protocol [7, 8]

The protocol consists of the main protocol document along with various annexures such as the budget sheet, curriculum vitae of investigators, the informed consent form, the investigators' brochure, and the case record form.

The protocol document should include the following information:

Title of the Study

This allows readers (and reviewers and funding agencies) to get an initial idea of what the study is about. While short and catchy titles are easy to remember, longer titles are more informative.

Protocol Version Number and Date

The version number and date are updated as amendments are made and help to ensure that all parties are using the same version of the protocol, and that the most recent version is in use.

Investigators and Sites

The names of all investigators along with degrees, affiliations, and contact details should be included. The principal investigator should be identified and the roles and responsibilities of all investigators specified. This information helps in the following ways:

- It gives credibility to the study if established researchers are part of the team.
- It allows delegation of responsibility among investigators.
- In multicenter studies, it gives ethics committees and funding agencies information about the magnitude of the study and the various collaborations.
- It helps reviewers to contact investigators for any clarifications.
- It helps to decide authorship for the final manuscript.

Project Summary

For lengthy protocols, a brief 250–300-word synopsis summarizing all the elements of the protocol may be included.

Introduction/Background

This is similar to the introduction section of a research paper. It gives the rationale for conducting the study and outlines the need for the study in the context of existing knowledge. This section should contain a summary of the problem that needs to be studied, a brief review of the available evidence, and a statement regarding the expected impact of the proposed study and how it will fill the gap in knowledge. The introduction should be concise and should include only relevant references without unnecessary historical details.

Hypothesis

A research hypothesis is a statement of expectation or prediction that will be tested by the research. The study hypothesis states what the researcher expects to find at the end of the study. It is often stated as a null hypothesis.

Objectives

The objectives are specific questions that the study aims to answer as opposed to goals which are broad statements of what the study hopes to achieve. The objectives of the study, classified as primary and secondary, should be outlined clearly.

Methodology

This is an important part of the protocol and should include details of the research design, the study setting, the research subjects, interventions, and the observations to be made.

A. *Study design*: The validity of study results depends on the study design. The design of the study (for example, descriptive, observational or experimental; prospective or retrospective; randomized or not; parallel-group or cross-over; type of control, if any; number of study arms) should be specified.
B. *Study setting*: This section should indicate where the study will be carried out (the center(s) where the study will be conducted, out-patient departments or wards; number of centers; number of countries).
C. *Research participants*: Inclusion and exclusion criteria for the study should be outlined. This should include details such as age, gender, physical status, and comorbidities. Exclusion criteria should not be stated as the converse of inclusion criteria, but should be specific conditions which will be excluded from the study.
D. *Details of screening and accrual*: The process of identifying potentially eligible participants and obtaining informed consent (including who will obtain consent,

and when and where) should be mentioned. Screening tools and baseline measurements should be enumerated. Details on refusals and non-eligible participants should be kept as part of the dataset.

E. *Allocation*: In experimental studies, details of how participants will be allotted to groups should be written. If the study is randomized, details of the technique of randomization and allocation concealment should be given, including who will be responsible for the randomization. If strata are planned during randomization, these should be pre-specified.

F. *Study interventions*: Complete details of interventions in both the control and the study arm(s) must be presented. Measures taken to prevent bias such as blinding of study personnel and participants or the use of dummies should be mentioned.

G. *Concomitant treatments*: Details of what other treatments will be allowed/prohibited during the study should be clearly specified.

H. *Data collection*: This includes the type of data to be collected (clinical/laboratory/radiology), by whom it will be collected, and at what time points. While standard procedures do not need detailing, any new procedure or technique must be explained in detail. If questionnaires are used, then a copy must be included in the protocol along with any translated versions. If assessors are blinded to treatment allocation, this must be specified.

I. *Outcomes and outcome measures*: Primary and secondary outcomes should be based on the corresponding study objectives and the measures which will be used to assess these outcomes should be specified.

J. *Follow-up*: any planned follow-up for efficacy/safety outcomes should be enumerated along with details of the frequency and duration of visits and expected data collection at each visit.

Safety and Adverse Event Reporting

A description of adverse events anticipated during the study should be listed along with expected frequency of occurrence. The guidelines for reporting of adverse events must be outlined (e.g., which terminology will be used, timelines for reporting). Rules for stopping the trial or withdrawing participants in case of adverse events must be laid down. If safety analysis is planned as part of the results, then the dataset which will be used (e.g., all participants who receive at least one dose of study medication) should be specified.

Statistical Plan

A. *Sample size*: The total sample size for the study and how this number was arrived at, including the number to be recruited at each center, should be specified. The feasibility of accruing the required number of patients and the expected duration of the study should be mentioned.

B. *Statistical analysis*: This section describes the statistical test(s) which will be used to analyze results. Details of the software to be used for statistical analysis should also be mentioned. The dataset which will be used for analysis (intention-to-treat, per-protocol) should be specified. If additional subgroup analyses are planned, details should be provided. The plan for any interim analysis, along with details of stopping rules, should be outlined. Level of significance, adjustments for multiple comparisons, and handling of missing data should be clarified.

Data Handling and Record Keeping

This section outlines details of how data will be recorded, stored, and monitored for quality assurance. A statement on how confidentiality of data will be maintained should be included.

References

The protocol must include references to original articles in the order in which they appear.

Glossary

This section of the protocol should provide definitions of important abbreviations, terms, and procedures which will be used during the study. Further information about the research protocol can be found in Chap. 5.

Ethical Considerations

All commonly expected risks and benefits to the participant should be enumerated. It should be specified that the study will be conducted in accordance with the principles of good clinical research practice. Information should be included on how informed consent will be obtained and how participant confidentiality will be maintained. Details of compensation which will be provided to study participants (if any) should be mentioned. This would include compensation for study-related procedures (time spent in hospital visits, travel costs) and compensation for research-related injury. Chapter 6 is dedicated on ethical considerations.

Dissemination of Results and Publication Policy

The protocol should specify how study findings will be shared including the names of authors who will be involved in publishing the results. Chapter 10 describes in detail the dissemination of results and publications policy.

Annexures to the Main Protocol Document

A. *Budget*: The total budget for the study with an item-wise and time-wise breakdown should be provided. This should include a budget justification.
B. *Funding*: This section includes details of funding received for the study along with contact details of the funding agency.
C. *Insurance*: If the study is covered by an insurance policy, details should be given.
D. *Curriculum vitae*: A brief curriculum vitae of all study personnel with details of qualifications, research training, and research experience should be attached to the protocol.
E. *Flowcharts*: Flow diagrams depicting the trial schema with timing of visits and data to be captured at each visit should be provided for easy understanding.
F. *Informed consent form*: Informed consent is defined as "a process by which a subject voluntarily confirms his or her willingness to participate in a particular trial, after having been informed of all aspects of the trial that are relevant to the subject's decision to participate" [7]. The informed consent form consists of the patient information sheet which outlines details of the trial which are necessary for the participant to make a decision to participate and the actual consent form which contains the signature of the participant/witness/legally acceptable representative and the investigator with the date. The patient information sheet should be written in simple, non-technical language and should be made available in all local languages commonly used at the sites where the study is to be conducted. Various guidelines are available which lay down certain key requirements of the patient information sheet [7, 9].
G. *Investigators' brochure*: As per ICH GCP guidelines, the investigators' brochure (IB) is defined as "A compilation of the clinical and nonclinical data on the investigational product(s) which is relevant to the study of the investigational product(s) in human subjects" [7]. The IB contains all information available that is relevant to the stage of clinical development of the investigational product. This includes data regarding physical, chemical and pharmaceutical properties and formulation, data from non-clinical studies (including pharmacology, pharmacokinetics, metabolism, and toxicology), and data from studies in humans (including pharmacokinetics, metabolism, pharmacodynamics, dose response, safety, efficacy, and marketing experience).
H. *Case report form*: This is a "printed, optical, or electronic document designed to record all of the protocol required information to be reported to the sponsor on each trial subject" [7].

Case report forms (CRFs) can be of two types: electronic (eCRF) or paper. The advantages of eCRF include [8, 10]:

- Elimination of the need to enter data from paper CRFs—thereby minimizing transcription errors.
- The ability to access data real-time.

- Ease of remote monitoring.
- Removal of the need to store paper CRFs.
- Early analysis of data and ability to provide early answers to queries.

However, the following factors need to be taken into account while planning eCRFs

- Availability of technology.
- Set-up costs.
- Computer literacy of the principal investigator and trial co-ordinator.
- Need for provision of an audit trail.
- Compliance with federal regulations. For example, in the USA, Title 21 Code of Federal Regulations (CFR) part 11 deals with requirements for software and systems involved in processing electronic data [11].

CRFs should collect all data that are needed for assessment (efficacy or safety) in a logical fashion which will facilitate data entry into the data management system [8]. Open-ended questions should be limited; instead, answer options (either lists or drop-down) should be provided. Each CRF should have a version number and date which should be updated if there are any changes in the CRF.

Research Team: Composition, Roles, and Responsibility

Composition of a Research Team

Most research is done using an interdisciplinary and multidisciplinary research team. Even if the research project is small, a single individual will find it difficult to run the entire project alone. It is therefore important to identify collaborators at an early stage. The team building should ideally start at the time the project is conceptualized. As the protocol is written, the research team can be further strengthened depending upon the various disciplines required for the study. It is important to bear in mind that collaborators do not necessarily have to be academics. It is equally important to have the support and cooperation of other staff like nurses, trial coordinators, statisticians, laboratory personnel, etc. However, all the staff involved in patient care need not be on the research team.

To be able to identify members who should be included in the team, the research question needs to be considered and the following questions need to be answered:

- Who is needed for conceptualizing and designing the study protocol?
- Who is needed to identify patients, help in obtaining consent and data collection?
- Who will perform the interventions/procedures defined in the protocol?
- Who will analyze the data?

Depending on the answers, colleagues and personnel can be approached to participate in the protocol.

Roles and Responsibilities

Most Institutional Review Boards will ask you to specify the roles and responsibilities of the team members at the time of submission of the project for review. This is an important step to ensure the optimum functioning of the study team. It includes creating a good working atmosphere, defining roles and responsibilities of each team member, and addressing issues of data collection, usage, and authorship.

Most study teams will have one or multiple investigators, a data manager, a trial coordinator, a research nurse and, sometimes, a research fellow. There may also be other team members like a pharmacist, a statistician, etc. as part of the research team. The roles and responsibilities of each of these members should be well-defined.

A. *Investigator*: A study may have one or many investigators. When there is more than one investigator, one is designed as Principal Investigator (PI). The other investigators are called co-investigators or sub-investigators. The PI is primarily responsible for conducting the study ethically and as per protocol. Managing the funds and their appropriate disbursement is the duty of the PI. Overall, the PI is like the captain of a ship and bears responsibility for the conduct of the entire study.
B. *Research Nurse*: The research nurse is a very strong asset to have on any research study. Due to their routine close interaction with patients, they are able to understand the needs and problems of patients accrued on the study. Besides the investigators, the only team member who can deal directly with the patients is a research nurse. The roles and responsibilities of a research nurse are vast. They include counseling and participation in informed consent, patient recruitment, collection and storage of tissue, and data collection.
C. *Data Manager*: As the name suggests, a data manager collects and maintains data on the study. Data managers generally do not have contact with patients and are not involved in the actual data collection from patients. The data obtained from the patients by the investigators or the research nurse are cleaned, collated, and entered into a pre-established database by the data manager. The data manager is responsible for formulating and implementing correct data management policies.

Obtaining Research Grants/Funding

Research funding is important to cover costs incurred during the study such as supplies, equipment, laboratory tests, travel, and salaries for personnel. Funding is also important for training research assistants and procurement of equipment which can help in local capacity-building.

Sources of Research Funding

The main sources of research funding are:

A. *Institutional departments or universities*—These usually have the capacity to assist small-scale studies. However, researchers at an early stage of their career may not be eligible for this type of funding.
B. *Government agencies*: Examples of these would include the National Institutes of Health (NIH) in the USA, the Medical Research Council (MRC) in the UK, and the Indian Council of Medical Research (ICMR). Such agencies may look specifically at the impact of the research on local health issues.
C. *Foundations/Charities*: e.g., the Bill and Melinda Gates foundation in the US and the Wellcome Trust in the UK. Charities and foundations usually have focused areas of interest for research.
D. *Commercial*: Pharmaceutical companies often sponsor large multi-centric studies; however, industry funding may lead to conflicts of interest and issues over dissemination of study results and intellectual property, and these issues must be discussed and documented in the protocol.

   More information on funding is found in Chap. 8.

Key Steps in Obtaining Research Funding

The steps in obtaining funding for research include:

A. Identify an organization which will be interested in supporting the planned research.
B. Review the criteria and guidelines for funding, including instructions for application.
C. Submit a proposal outlining the background, objectives, methodology, budget, and research implications with a detailed budget sheet. Some funding agencies may require a "pre-proposal," which is a brief summary of the project and is used by the agency as an initial tool to identify projects which are then evaluated in detail [12].
D. Projects which are identified as being potentially suitable for funding are then sent for peer review to assess the merits of the study and the suitability for funding.

What Are the Factors That Impact on Research Funding?

Reviewers rate various parameters of protocols which are submitted for funding [12–15]:

A. *The research question*: Does the project ask a new and focused question? Is the research important and relevant to the community?

B. *The research methods*: Is the methodology appropriate and feasible? Is the time scale realistic? Are there any ethical or regulatory concerns?
C. *The research team*: Is the research team capable of carrying out the research successfully?
   Do individual researchers have previous research experience? What is their publication record? Have they successfully obtained other grants?

D. *The research setting*: Does the institute have the infrastructure to support the research in terms of space, equipment, laboratory facilities, and mentors?
E. *The research budget*: Is the budget appropriate and realistic? Is everything that is budgeted for really needed? Is the budget adequate to cover the costs of the trial?

What Can Researchers Do to Improve Their Chances of Being Funded [12, 13]?

- The project: Ask a clear and relevant question. Make the protocol precise and easy to read.
- The budget: Keep it rational and not overly ambitious.
- Collaborate: with other researchers who have previous research and funding experience in the same field.
- Improve their curriculum vitae by publishing in the area of interest.
- Confirm that the agency they are approaching is interested in funding that type of research.
- Follow instructions for submitting funding proposals.
- Use reviewers' comments constructively and re-frame the proposal accordingly.

Conduct of the Study: Data Management, Monitoring, and Analysis

Once the research protocol is finalized and approved by the IRB and funding for the research has been obtained, it is time to begin the study. During the study, it is essential that investigators [9]:

- Adhere to the protocol
- Maintain ethics
- Objectively measure outcomes
- Record observations appropriately
- Conduct suitable data analysis to give valid results
- Present the results to others

The following key steps are crucial to the successful conduct of a research study.

Trial Registration [9, 15–18]

Trial registration refers to the publication of an internationally agreed set of information about the design, conduct, and administration of clinical trials. These details are published on a publicly accessible website managed by a registry conforming to standards. Trial registration is important for ethical and scientific reasons and must be done before the first subject is recruited.

Trial registration serves the following purposes:

A. Ensures that the public has information about ongoing and completed research studies.
B. Identifies missing gaps in research.
C. Promotes efficient allocation of research funds.
D. Ensures that researchers adhere to the protocol during the course of the research study.
E. Allows early identification of problems in the research methodology.
F. Provides researchers, reviewers, and editors the background for understanding the study results.
G. Promotes collaboration.
H. Reduces publication bias and selective reporting by alerting researchers to studies that have not been published.
I. Avoids duplication of research.

The World Health Organization International Clinical Trials Registry platform receives data from several independent data registries [17]. Researchers can register their trial in any of the individual registries in this platform or in any other registry approved by the International Council of Medical Journal Editors.

Investigators Training [10]

For multi-center trials and for single-center trials in which multiple investigators are participating, it is important to ensure that there is standardization of trial procedures. Investigators may therefore need to be trained and provided with a list of standard operating procedures (SOPs) before the trial commences. Training could include various aspects such as subject accrual, protocol procedures, good clinical practice, completing CRFs, sample collection and storage, and adverse event reporting.

Essential Documents and Master File [7, 10]

The trial master file containing all essential documents needed for the conduct of the trial should be organized prior to commencing the study. Patient-specific information which can reveal treatment allocation should not be stored in the master file.

The master file helps in: (a) the orderly conduct of the trial; (b) proving compliance with GCP; (c) allowing easy monitoring and auditing; and, (d) providing a ready reference for investigators.

For multi-center trials, each center should have an investigator site file which contains documents specific to the site.

Site Initiation [10, 19, 20]

The site-initiation meeting is conducted to verify that all trial-related documents and materials are in place and ensures that all study personnel understand the actual processes involved in the conduct of the study. Once the site is initiated, recruitment of patients can commence. For multi-center sponsored studies, a clinical research associate (CRA) appointed by the sponsor conducts the trial site initiation. For investigator-initiated studies, the meeting can be conducted by the study personnel.

Recruitment of Patients

Recruitment is probably the most challenging aspect of the study. It is important to meet recruitment goals to ensure that the study is completed within budget and without delay. In addition to enlisting participants from the hospital population, patient recruitment can be accelerated by approaching other medical practitioners and through advertisements (after prior approval from the Institutional Ethics Committee).

Screening and Enrolment

A log of all patients who meet the eligibility criteria for participation should be maintained (screening log) along with a list of patients who are finally enrolled, documenting the reasons for non-participation (screen failures). The CONSORT guidelines for reporting of results of clinical trials mandate that this information should be reported in the form of a participant flowchart [20]. This ensures that ineligible patients are not enrolled and exposed to harm, documents absence of a selection bias in patient recruitment, and helps readers to assess the generalizability of the study results. Informed consent is obtained from enrolled participants by a member of the research team and the process is documented in the source document, with a copy of the informed consent document given to the participant.

Study Activities

Once consent has been obtained, study procedures commence and the participant can be randomized to receive study interventions. Assessment of efficacy and safety outcomes is performed as per the protocol and SOPs.

Protocol Deviations and Amendments

In any clinical trial, there may be instances of non-compliance with the study protocol. This may occur due to various reasons: the investigator deviates from the protocol to ensure participant safety, the participant does not comply with the protocol, or other unanticipated extraneous factors. A protocol deviation is defined as "any change, divergence, or departure from the study design or procedures defined in the protocol" [21]. Important protocol deviations (sometimes referred to as violations) are "a subset of protocol deviations that may significantly impact the completeness, accuracy, and/or reliability of the study data or that may significantly affect a subject's rights, safety, or well-being" [21].

The ICH-GCP has defined guidelines regarding documentation and reporting of protocol deviations [21].

Safety Reporting [7]

ICH GCP has standard definitions for "adverse events" (AES) and "serious adverse events" (SAEs) during a clinical trial. While SAEs should be reported to the sponsor and the IRB within stipulated timelines, reporting of AEs is usually done on an annual basis at the time of the study review.

Monitoring

Is defined as "The act of overseeing the progress of a clinical trial, and of ensuring that it is conducted, recorded, and reported in accordance with the protocol, SOPs, GCP, and the applicable regulatory requirement(s)" [7].

Monitoring is necessary to ensure that:

- The rights and well-being of participants are protected.
- Trial data are accurate, verifiable from source documents and complete.
- The conduct of the trial is as per protocol and in accordance with the principles of GCP and with applicable regulatory requirements [7].

The extent and frequency of monitoring is proportional to the size, complexity, risks, and duration of the trial. Usually, the plan for monitoring is pre-specified in the study protocol. In sponsored trials, a clinical research associate (CRA) affiliated to the contract research organisation (CRO) carries out the monitoring. In investigator-initiated studies, the investigator may consider employing an independent person to carry out the same task.

The purpose of the monitoring visit is to: [7, 10]

- Check whether recruitment is on schedule.
- Verify adherence to the protocol and identify deviations.
- Review CRFs and cross-check data with source documents.
- Check investigational product management and accountability.
- Confirm adverse event reporting.
- Ensure that all documentation is up-to-date [7, 10].

Data Management and Analysis

Data should be entered into a database on a real-time basis, minimizing the delay between data collection and data entry. This helps to:

- Discover errors in the data collection process early.
- Reduce the possibility of loss of data.
- Allow better tracking of progress of the study.
- Allow easy verification of data from source documents in case of queries [19].

To minimize errors, data entry is sometimes done independently by two people (double data entry) and any discrepancies are then corrected. The database is scanned periodically to identify missing or unlikely values and is then cleaned by sending these queries to individual site coordinators. Special statistical techniques are available to deal with missing data. Statistical analysis is carried out using the tests specified in the protocol and the study results are generated. Chapter …gives detailed information on statistical analysis and data management.

Study Completion and Site Close-Out [10]

Once follow-up of the last participant is over, or in some cases, if the study is terminated prematurely, the study can be closed at that site. At the time of site closure, it should be ensured that any data queries/clarifications are resolved, unused drugs are returned to the sponsor or destroyed as per policy, and the study report is finalized and sent to the sponsor. The IRB should receive the study closure report along with a summary of the results.

Scientific Writing

Publishing the research findings is as important a component of the study as conducting the research—the impact of good research would be negligible if it is not translated into a research paper. Articles published in journals help for a wider dissemination of the study results, thus making them applicable to larger populations. Also, research that is not published is not considered as evidence and cannot be put into clinical practice. If the protocol is well-written, the process of scientific writing becomes simpler and easier.

The steps of writing a research paper include:

Writing an Outline

The first step in writing a research paper would be to construct an outline comprising the points that need to be highlighted in the paper. The outline helps to put down all the important ideas, irrespective of their order. This will help in building a template for the paper and prevent missing out on important study results. The outline should broadly define the topic, the need for conducting the study, the major findings, and the conclusion.

Preparing the First Draft

The first draft of the paper is the first structured version of the scientific paper. It should include subheadings like Introduction, Materials and Methods, Results, Discussion (the IMRaD format), and Conclusions. Once the first draft is ready, it is advisable to identify the target journal/s to which the paper will be submitted. It is also be prudent to discuss the draft with coauthors, guides, teachers, or peers. It is important to include coauthors (along with specific tasks and responsibilities for each coauthor) and peers early in the writing of a scientific paper so that their suggestions and inputs can be incorporated into the paper.

Construction of the Final Paper

This step involves the detailed writing of each section of the paper using all the available inputs and an idea of the target journal. It may help to start with the materials and methods and results sections as these detail the factual aspects of the paper. These are relatively easy to write as compared to the introduction and discussion sections, which require some creative writing.

It is important at this step to include everything that is relevant to the paper into the various sections. It is often useful to write the initial drafts without editing as this may interrupt the chain of thought, which is important for the smooth flow of ideas.

The intent and application of each of the subsections should be understood in advance. Outlined below is the brief summary of the intent of each of the common subsections in a research paper.

A. *Abstract*: The abstract presents a summary of the research findings as well as the rationale, description, and results of the study at a quick glance. Readers should be able to identify interest in the paper by reading the abstract.
B. *Introduction*: This section should introduce the concept and rationale of the research hypothesis, the need for the research, and a brief comment on the existing literature on the topic. The aims and objectives should be clearly defined towards the end of this section.
C. *Materials and Methods*: The aim of this section is to enable readers to understand the exact characteristics of the study population, the procedures that have been carried out, and the methodology for documenting the results. This will help in the application of the results of the study to actual clinical practice by the readers. The different statistical methods used to assess the results should be outlined in this section.
D. *Results*: This section describes and illustrates the results of the study. It is the most objective and factual part of the paper. There should be no attempt made to discuss the results of the paper in this section. Liberal use of tables and figures may help to simplify the information.
E. *Discussion*: The objective of this section is to discuss the results and compare them to available literature in a manner that will lead to the conclusion derived from the research. The discussion part of the paper puts the results of the study in the context of existing and prior knowledge of the subject. Enumerating and discussing the limitations of the study is an important part of this section.

Editing and Formatting

This is the final and crucial stage of scientific writing prior to submission. The manuscript should be edited to ensure information is presented accurately and concisely. Verbose or flowery descriptions are not appreciated by most journals. It is important to economize on the number of words without changing the meaning of the results. During editing, the specific instructions to authors provided by each journal should be considered. The entire manuscript (tables, figures, and references included) should be prepared as per these instructions. This cannot be overemphasized. There are several guidelines for writing scientific papers depending on the type of research study including CONSORT (for randomized trials) [20], PRISMA (for systematic reviews and meta-analyses) [22], STROBE (for observational studies) [23], and MOOSE (for systematic reviews and meta-analyses of observational studies) [24].

Ethics of Scientific Writing

Plagiarism is not tolerated in the scientific writing community. All information cited from others' research has to be adequately referenced. Even if referenced, direct quotation from texts is generally not acceptable. Most journals use specialized software for plagiarism checks. The consequences of finding a plagiarized manuscript are grave, putting into jeopardy all further research from that particular group of researchers and their institution.

Summary

In this chapter, the process of clinical research has been described in depth. While the research idea itself involves much of the innovative aspect of research, it is important for the process to be systematically followed for a successful research project. It is key to understand that what is important is not whether a study is "positive" or "negative," but the fact that the research question is reliably answered, regardless of whether the hypothesis is proved or disproved.

References

1. Campbell JD. Formulating the research question. 2015. https://www.atsu.edu/research/pdfs/campbell_syllabus.pdf. Accessed 1 Feb 2015.
2. Thabane L, Thomas T, Ye C, Paul J. Posing the research question: not so simple. Can J Anaesth. 2009;56:71–9.
3. Bragge P. Asking good clinical research questions and choosing the right study design. Injury. 2010;41:S3–6.
4. Clouse RE. Proposing a good research question: a simple formula for success. Gastrointest Endosc. 2005;61:279–80.
5. Stillwell SB, Fineout-Overholt E, Melnyk BM, Williamson KM. Evidence-based practice, step by step: asking the clinical question: a key step in evidence-based practice. Am J Nurs. 2010;110:58–61.
6. Pubmed Tutorial. Bethesda (MD): National Library of Medicine (US) 2001. Updated 2013 Sept 20. www.nlm.nih.gov/bsd/disted/pubmedtutorial/020_350.html. Accessed 1 Feb 2015.
7. ICH Expert Working Group. ICH harmonized tripartite guideline: guideline for good clinical practice E6 (R1). International Conference on Harmonisation (ICH); 1996 June 10. http://www.ich.org/fileadmin/Public_Web_Site/ICH_Products/Guidelines/Efficacy/E6_R1/Step4/E6_R1__Guideline.pdf. Accessed 1 Feb 2015.

8. Chin R, Lee BY, editors. Principles and practice of clinical trial medicine. Amsterdam: Elsevier/Academic Press; 2008.
9. Fathalla MF. A practical guide for health researchers. WHO Regional Publications, Eastern Mediterranean Series; 30. Cairo; 2004. http://www.emro.who.int/publications/pdf/healthresearchers_guide.pdf. Accessed 1 Feb 2015.
10. Chin R, Bairu M, editors. Global clinical trials: effective implementation and management. Amsterdam: Elsevier/Academic Press; 2011.
11. US Department of Health and Human Services. Food and Drug Administration. Center for Drug Evaluation and Research (CDER). Center for Biologics Evaluation and Research (CBER). Guidance for industry. Part 11, electronic records; electronic signatures—scope and application [Internet]. 2003 Aug. http://www.fda.gov/downloads/RegulatoryInformation/Guidances/ucm125125.pdf. Accessed 1 Feb 2015.
12. Eastwood PR, Naughton MT, Calverley P, Zeng G, Beasley R, Robinson B, Lee YC. How to write research papers and grants: 2011 Asian Pacific Society for Respirology Annual Scientific Meeting Postgraduate Session. Respirology. 2012;17:792–801.
13. Chan JK, Shalhoub J, Gardiner MD, Suleman-Verjee L, Nanchahal J. Strategies to secure surgical research funding: fellowships and grants. JRSM Open. 2014;5:1–5.
14. Grants and funding. National Institutes of Health office of extramural research. Updated 2014 Aug 12. Accessed 1 February 2015.
15. Zarin DA, Keselman A. Registering a clinical trial in ClinicalTrials.gov. Chest. 2007;31: 909–12.
16. About ClinicalTrials.gov. US National Institutes of Health. Reviewed 2014 May. https://clinicaltrials.gov/ct2/about-site. Accessed 1 Feb 2015.
17. World Health Organization. International Clinical Trials Registry Platform. Geneva: World Health Organization. Updated 2015. http://www.who.int/ictrp/en/. Accessed 1 Feb 2015.
18. World Medical Association Declaration of Helsinki. Ethical principles for medical research involving human subjects. 1964 June (Updated Oct 2008). http://www.wma.net/en/30publications/10policies/b3/17c.pdf. Accessed 1 Feb 2015.
19. Step-by-step guide to doing Clinical Research—a methodological approach. AO foundation. 2015. https://www.aofoundation.org/Structure/research/clinical-research/step-guide-clinical-research/doing/Pages/doing.aspx. Accessed 1 Feb 2015.
20. Schulz KF, Altman DG, Moher D, CONSORT Group. CONSORT 2010 statement: updated guidelines for reporting parallel group randomized trials. Ann Intern Med. 2010;152:726–32.
21. ICH. E3 implementation working group ICH E3 guideline: structure and content of clinical study reports questions & answers 7 June 2012. 2015. http://www.ich.org/fileadmin/Public_Web_Site/ICH_Products/Guidelines/Efficacy/E3/E3_Q_As_Step4.pdf 3. Accessed 1 Feb 2015.
22. Moher D, Liberati A, Tetzlaff J, Altman DG, PRISMA Group. Preferred reporting items for systematic reviews and meta-analyses: the PRISMA statement. Ann Intern Med. 2009;151: 264–9.
23. Vandenbroucke JP, von Elm E, Altman DG, Gøtzsche PC, Mulrow CD, Pocock SJ, Poole C, Schlesselman JJ, Egger M, STROBE Initiative. Strengthening the Reporting of Observational Studies in Epidemiology (STROBE): Explanation and elaboration. Int J Surg. 2014;12: 1500–24.
24. Stroup DF, Berlin JA, Morton SC, Olkin I, Williamson GD, Rennie D, Moher D, Becker BJ, Sipe TA, Thacker SB. Meta-analysis of observational studies in epidemiology: a proposal for reporting. Meta-analysis of Observational Studies in Epidemiology (MOOSE) group. JAMA. 2000;283:2008–12.

Chapter 3
Types of Research Designs

Fedor Moissenko, Cornelia Braicu, Ciprian Tomuleasa,
and Ioana Berindan-Neagoe

Abstract The research design can be defined as the plan of action to be followed to answer the research question. The type of question dictates the type of study design. Primary research is research which seeks to obtain new data about the phenomena studied, while secondary research is the research which analyses the data and results of studies already done.

The types of research can be classified as quantitative (correlational, comparative, experimental, etc.) or qualitative.

The quantitative studies can be classified as cross-sectional, "before and after," longitudinal. A time classification will group them into retrospective, prospective, and both (retrospective and prospective). Depending on the nature of the investigation, the types of research could be also classified as descriptive, comparative, or experimental.

The qualitative research includes the phenomenological, ethnographic, historical, case studies, grounded theory.

Secondary research includes systematic, narrative, and meta-analysis reviews.

Keywords Types of research • Designs • Quantitative • Qualitative • Primary • Secondary

---

This chapter tries to illustrate the concept that each research question is best answered by a certain type of study, in a set of given circumstances.

F. Moissenko, M.D., Ph.D. (✉)
Laboratory of Nanobiotechnology, St. Petersburg Academic University—
Nanotechnology Research and Education Center of the Russian Academy of Sciences,
8/3 Khlopina Street, St. Petersburg, NA 194021, Russia
e-mail: moiseenkofv@gmail.com

C. Braicu
Research Center for Functional Genomics, Biomedicine and Translational Medicine,
"Iuliu Hatieganu" University of Medicine and Pharmacy, Victor Babes, Cluj-Napoca,
Romania
e-mail: braicucornelia@yahoo.com; cornelia.braicu@umfcluj.ro

C. Tomuleasa, M.D., Ph.D. • I. Berindan-Neagoe, Ph.D.
Research Center for Functional Genomics and Translational Medicine, Iuliu Hatieganu
University of Medicine and Pharmacy, Cluj Napoca, Cluj 400020, Romania
e-mail: ciprian.tomuleasa@umfcluj.ro; Ioana.neagoe@umfcluj.ro

© Springer International Publishing Switzerland 2016
D.C. Stefan (ed.), *Cancer Research and Clinical Trials
in Developing Countries*, DOI 10.1007/978-3-319-18443-2_3

What Is Research?

The definition of **research** [1] is that of a *systematic investigation/inquiry* that includes research development, hypotheses testing, and evaluation of data, designed to develop or contribute to generalizable knowledge, and pose new questions for future research to explore.

A *systematic inquiry* should meet the following criteria [2]:

- One or more research questions are formulated and an attempt is made to find the corresponding answers.
- A methodology is followed in the collection of data.
- The data obtained are analyzed by either quantitative or qualitative methods.
- The results of the analysis are synthesized in conclusions (which contribute to generalizable knowledge).

As a result, research consists of:

- Asking a question that nobody has asked before
- Doing the necessary work to find the answer
- Communicating the knowledge to a larger audience

In practice, research methods vary widely, depending on the academic discipline's accepted standards, the individual researcher's preferences, or a particular study's needs. Research in science often involves conducting experiments in the laboratory or in the field.

Research is not a solitary activity, but an act of community. As a member of the research community, you are building on the knowledge that others have acquired before you and providing a road map for those who come after you. You are adding to a body of work that will never be complete. Research is an ongoing, collaborative process with no finish line in sight.

Research Is Conducted According to the Scientific Method

The scientific method is a way to ask and answer scientific questions by making observations and doing experiments. Scientific methods help scientists study how nature and the environment work.

The steps involved in scientific method [3] are outlined below:

- From observations and existing information on a subject, a problem is identified. A research question emerges as the problem is analyzed.
- A hypothesis is constructed which aims to answer the question.
- The hypothesis is tested by designing and conducting an experiment or collecting information related to it.
- The expected results (which would confirm the hypothesis) are compared with the observed results.

- A conclusion is drawn: either (a) the hypothesis is not confirmed and further refinement of it—or of the experiment—is necessary; or, (b) the hypothesis is confirmed.
- The conclusions are communicated; further research may be conducted on the basis of the new findings.

It is important for the experiment to be a "fair test." A fair test occurs when you change only one factor (variable) and keep all other conditions the same—i.e., adjusting for possible confounding factors. In practice, for biological and medical experiments in particular, this requirement is unlikely to be achieved and at best the number of investigational variables/factors is kept to a minimum.

The Importance of the Research Question

A research question presents the idea to be investigated in a study and provides the essential focus of the research. A well-written research question will also shed light on appropriate research methods (e.g., specify the intended actions of the variables and how an experimental intervention might be measured) [4].

Characteristics of a good research question are:

- It is specific.
- It is clear.
- It refers to the **problem or phenomenon**.
- It reflects the intervention in experimental research.
- It notes the target group of participants.

Types of Research Design

The research design can be defined as the plan of action to be followed to answer the research question. As shown in Table 3.1, the type of question dictates the type of study design. Following a specific, previously verified and standardized plan of action in research ensures that the results obtained correspond to reality.

This section will describe the characteristics of various types of research designs, their usage, type of output, and limitations. The reader should keep in mind that the classification presented is based on methodology and not on the area of application. The same methodology, i.e., the same type of design, may apply to solving questions about a large number of diverse phenomena.

To start, it is important to distinguish between primary research, which seeks to obtain new data about the phenomena studied, and secondary research, which analyses the data and results of studies already done. Both categories will be described in the following pages.

Table 3.1 Examples of research questions: each type of question is best answered by a certain type of research (derived from Haber J. Chap. 2, Table 2.2) [4]

Example	Format	Research type
		Quantitative
Is there a relationship between ever smoking cannabis and cancer development in adults over the age of 50?	Is there a relationship between X (independent variable) and Y (dependent variable) in the specified population?	Correlational
Do people who eat healthy diets and engage in physical activity have better cancer survival rates than those who do not eat healthy diets and engage in physical activity?	Is there a difference in Y (dependent variable) between people who have X characteristics (independent variable) and those who do not have X characteristics?	Comparative
Is there a difference in 5-year survival in stage II breast cancer patients who received tamoxifen versus those who did not receive it?	Is there a difference in Y (dependent variable) between Group A, who received X (independent variable) and Group B who did not receive X?	Experimental
		Qualitative
How did breast cancer affect the breast cancer survivors' family dynamics, as well as their social and cultural well-being?	What is/was it like to have X?	Phenomenological

Primary Research

If the data obtained are measurable and expressed in figures, the study type falls under the category of quantitative research. Other studies may target phenomena that cannot be measured—like emotions or opinions—and such research is therefore qualitative. Sometimes both qualitative and quantitative methods may be used in a study. For instance, a study which describes a chemical reaction can be qualitative if it describes only the reactants and the substances resulting from their interaction, and quantitative if it measures the amount of resulting product as a function of temperature.

Quantitative Designs

This description follows the classification proposed by Kumar [5]. The quantitative designs may be grouped according to:

- The number of contacts with the study population (i.e., a group of individual entities entered in the study: humans, animals, plants, bacteria, etc.)
- The reference period: an investigation in the past or a planned follow-up in the future.

– The nature of the investigation: is it observational only or does it include an intervention?

1. *According to the <u>number of contacts with the study population</u>, designs may be:*

   (a) *Cross-sectional.* This type of design investigates a whole population or a representative sample of it, at a given moment in time, in order to determine the prevalence of a certain phenomenon. An example of use for such a design: determining the prevalence of insomnia in people living within a radius of 3 km from a busy airport. The design requires that the population is identified, its members (or a sample of them) are contacted, and then asked about their sleep characteristics. Such studies cost little and the results are straightforward. The information is limited to a moment in time and does not necessarily connect the cause with an effect, unless the findings are compared with those obtained in a similar population which is not exposed to the presumptive cause. Many epidemiological studies utilize such a design.

   (b) *Before-and-after.* The cross-sectional design can be used to measure the change in the phenomenon studied after a certain period of time, if it is performed twice on the same population and with the same method of data collection, at the beginning and at the end of the time period. This type of "before and after" design is useful to evaluate the effect of an intervention applied after the first cross-sectional investigation. Considering the example described in (*a*), the intervention may be a flight interdiction between certain hours at night.

   In this broad category fall all the clinical trials, where patients with a particular disease receive a new treatment and the measure of outcome variable is measured before and after the intervention.

   (c) *Longitudinal.* A number of iterations of a cross-sectional study over a certain time period can provide information about the evolution of a phenomenon over time in the population studied. Extending the example given above, repeating the study several times over a year may find that initially the insomnia prevalence decreases but later it increases again, possibly due to rescheduling of late evening flights to the late afternoon, when the people are at home from work.

   Longitudinal studies may suffer from a *conditioning effect*: after a number of iterations of the study, the human subjects know what is expected of them, or simply lose interest in the study and their answers may not reflect reality. Generally, longitudinal studies are observational, aiming at finding correlations between various phenomena.

2. *According to the <u>reference period</u> a study which analyzes past events is retrospective while one which follows the phenomenon studied into the future is prospective. Both retrospective and prospective methods are sometimes used in the same investigation.*

   (a) *Retrospective.* This type of study looks for answers in the analysis of data recorded in the past or an analysis of people's recollections of past events.

As the information is readily available, the research requires relatively little time. However, as the data were not specifically recorded for the study purpose, they may often be incomplete. Also, it is often impossible to identify possible mistakes in the records. People's memories may also be incomplete or distorted.

Retrospective trials are usually valued less than prospective ones, even when medical records are considered to be objective. Another confounding factor, besides incomplete recorded information, might be investigator bias. For example: a retrospective comparison of the efficacy, in terms of overall survival, of two types of treatment for cancer—one more aggressive and the second less aggressive. The physicians tend to treat aggressively those patients who are in better overall condition. Yet they are not necessarily representative of the majority of patients. As a better overall condition is also an important prognostic factor for survival, the results of the study would be biased.

(b) *Prospective*. In this design, data collection starts at the onset of the study and continues for the planned duration of the research. This type of study may be used for evaluating the outcome of an intervention or an experiment, but also for assessing the effects in time, on a given population, of certain risk factors. The advantages of a prospective design include selecting the subjects, planning the intervention, and planned and supervised data collection.

(c) *Retrospective–prospective*. Here, instead of collecting the initial, baseline data at the onset of the study, already available data from the past are used. The effect of an experiment, intervention, or incidental event (an epidemic, for instance) is then studied prospectively.

3. *The <u>nature of the investigation</u> may be that of a mere observation of the various characteristics of the subject or of a group of subjects or may include a comparison between two or more groups of observed subjects, or even more, it may include an experiment.*

(a) *Descriptive studies*. Here the research question can be answered by observations and measurements which comprehensively characterize the subject (or group of subjects) investigated. No hypothesis is formulated relative to the research question and no intervention takes place. The observations are noted, quantified (when feasible), and analyzed. An example of such a study may be the description of a rare disease or of a newly discovered species. Case series studies fall mostly under this category.

Cohort studies are a particular type in this category, which consists of identifying and following up a group of people with a certain common characteristic. The common factor most of the time is a supposed risk factor (e.g., living within 10 km of a nuclear plant, in the path of the prevailing winds), but it may also be a neutral characteristic: year of birth, for instance. Cohort studies are prospective and data may be collected cross-sectionally or longitudinally. More than one possible outcome can be studied. The evidence for causality obtained from cohort studies is strong, but this design requires a large sample size and a long follow-up interval; these requirements translate to high costs [6].

(b) *Comparative studies*. In this design, data obtained about two different study subjects (such as microorganisms, objects, population groups, etc.) or about the same study subject at two different points in time are compared. Similarities or differences are identified; and, patterns or trends over time can be detected. Such observations may be analyzed to see if they support a hypothesis or not. An example would be to compare two viruses in order to see which one survives longer when left on a door handle.

(c) *Experimental studies*. The characteristic of experimental studies is that one variable (called "independent") is manipulated and the effect of this action on the subjects is measured. Variables which are presumed to be influenced by the experiment are called "dependent." All other factors which could possibly influence the effect of the independent variable have to be controlled: either kept constant or their action should be accounted for in evaluating the result of the experiment (such control is the condition of a "fair" test). This type of design is suitable for detecting causality and, in practice, is used to evaluate the effect of a treatment on a disease (see Chap. 8), the effect of a program on a population, etc. Experimental investigation can be done under numerous designs; a number of which are described below.

- The *after-only model* is, in fact, a retrospective–prospective design where the study starts immediately after the intervention considered as the experiment. Information of the status of the subjects studied before the intervention is obtained retrospectively while the data on the changes after the intervention are collected prospectively.

- If the study starts by obtaining a baseline status of the subjects by a cross-sectional inquiry before the intervention, and a second cross-sectional evaluation is done at a time when the intervention is expected to have produced results, that is a *before-and–after* design.

- *The controlled study*. The two designs described above can be used to assess the extent to which an intervention reduces or eliminates a condition already existing in the study population. However, when the intervention is meant to prevent the occurrence of a certain condition (for instance vaccination against an infectious disease), a *control group* is used. Such a design requires that two groups of subjects are formed, whose biological characteristics are similar; one group receives the intervention and the other is just observed. When the intervention is supposed to have produced its effects, the expected dependent variables are measured (in the case of a vaccine, the incidence of the infectious disease) in both groups and the differences are analyzed statistically to test their significance. Controlled groups are also useful, of course, for evaluating the efficacy of a new treatment versus the existing standard of care.

Ideally, controls should be *concurrent* but at times *historical controls* are used. Historical controls are better than no controls, but the design suffers from the shortcomings of any retrospective study.

At times, *patients can be their own controls*, which means that the study arms are identical. For instance, a patient with varicose ulcers on both legs may receive the test treatment on one leg and the standard treatment on the other leg.

Another method is that of *matched controls*, where for each case a control is chosen who matches all important variables.

It is often necessary to account for the *placebo effect* when testing a new treatment. It has been observed that, if the patient expects an improvement of his/her condition from a treatment, some change for the better will be noted even if the treatment doesn't work. The control arm should receive an inactive treatment that is similar in appearance to the real one, and if the improvement rates are similar, then the tested treatment is no better than placebo. This approach can be used only when no standard treatment already exists that is better than placebo.

An even more efficient comparison is possible by *blinding*: neither the patient nor the study personnel, including scientists, know which medication is the test one and which one is placebo. Blinding eliminates the possibility of subjectively ascribing better outcomes to the test medication, if it is known who received it.

- *The randomized controlled study.* The allocation of subjects to the intervention or non-intervention arms of the study may be biased if done by members of the study team. This can be overcome by randomization: patients are chosen to be part of one of the two groups, usually following random allocation generated by computer. In this way, each patient has the same probability of being allocated to any of the groups. Randomization contributes to making the *case* (i.e., subjects undergoing the intervention) and *control* groups more comparable, by avoiding the predominance of subjects with a particular characteristic in one of the arms.

  The randomized controlled study provides the strongest evidence on the causal relationship between two variables.

- *Clinical trials.* Mentioned here for completeness' sake, clinical trials are described in Chap. 4.

Qualitative Study Designs [7]

(a) *Phenomenological studies.* This type of study describes the "lived experiences" of the subjects who went through a particular event (for example: a hostage situation), with emphasis on the meaning of those experiences for the subject. The most frequently used method of investigation is the interview. The researcher needs to isolate his or her own thoughts or feelings on the event studied and not let them interfere with the interview process, in order to be able to record accurately the psychological reactions of the interviewee. This technique is called "bracketing."

(b) *Ethnographic studies.* Used mostly in anthropological research, ethnography deals with the cultural characteristics of a group. The researcher often goes to live with the particular group (such as the Amish people in the USA, for example) and notes their system of values, codes of behavior, the way they communicate, and so on. Interviews are done, with a number of individuals from the group ("key informants"), in order to obtain more specific data about certain cultural aspects. Bracketing may be necessary in order to understand the culture of the group better.

(c) *Grounded theory.* This design will be described here in a succinct manner and the reader is invited to consult the literature referred to here, for further details. Proposed by Glaser and Strauss in 1967 [8], this design consists of obtaining information around the research question by means of questionnaires administered in interviews. The information is analyzed in a specific manner, which is essential to this design, in order to generate a "substantive theory," meaning a coherent theory where each concept is "grounded" in the obtained data. This method avoids intuitive interpretation of data, which may be biased by the researcher's own experiences, knowledge, and mentality. An open mind is crucial to extracting the meaning from the interviews. For this reason, researchers would not consult the literature prior to collecting the data, but would do it after the analysis, to see whether their conclusions have also been published by others. This avoids abandoning the analysis once familiar themes are identified, thus neglecting possibly new, hitherto unknown aspects.

The data analysis takes place simultaneously with data collection. It consists of breaking the answers into elementary components (ideas, statements, and actions) and *coding* them for further reference. Comparisons are continually made between data, individual answers, and codes, with the purpose of extracting common themes but also of understanding the differences. Researchers write frequent memos about the individual interviews, which stimulates their ideation around the issues detected. The analysis may indicate new directions to investigate or gaps in the information, which are explored by new interviews and new questions. This approach constitutes *theoretical sampling.*

The substantive theory is constructed by connecting the codes in broader *categories* or *concepts* and further connecting the concepts. The theory is "grounded" because every code and concept can be traced back to the primary data [7, 9].

(d) *Historical studies.* This design is about identifying, retrieving, evaluating, and reporting data from the past. Historical sources are used: documents, graphic representations, monuments, oral histories, etc. These sources should satisfy the researcher that they are genuine and truthful in the way they reflect historic events.

(e) *Case studies.* These studies consist of an in-depth examination of companies, institutions, groups of people, diseases, laws, events, etc. Data are collected by observation, interviews (structured or not), analysis of documents, reports, or diaries. Themes and patterns are defined from the collected material ("*content analysis*").

(f) *Action research.* A type of research centers on finding "actions" which would improve work conditions and practices, following which the effects of applying the particular action are studied, is known as action research. The results of this type of study apply mostly to the setting where it was performed and are not necessarily generalizable [10].

Secondary Research

Narrative Review

This type of study offers a broad overview of the topic addressed, based on the literature, where the published studies are not selected or analyzed systematically, leaving room for a more subjective approach.

Systematic Review

A more structured approach is taken here: inclusion and exclusion criteria are established beforehand and enunciated in the published review. Efforts are made to find all published studies on the chosen subject. The analysis plan is also prepared in advance and presented to the reader. The methodology used in each study selected is evaluated for quality. The results are presented critically, trying to account for differences noted between studies.

Meta-Analysis

Taking a step further from the systematic review, a meta-analysis presents a quantitative summary of the results of various studies. When possible, a *pooled analysis* of the published data is presented. Odds ratios of various correlations found by the studies analyzed are often presented in *forest plots*. A meta-analysis of randomized controlled studies may confidently establish causal relationships between phenomena. Even stronger meta-analyses can be done by re-analyzing individual data and by prospectively performing studies with the same protocols, which in time provide large sets of perfectly comparable and analyzable data [11].

References

1. Code of Federal Regulations; Department of Health and Human Services. Protection of human subjects: Part 46. Section 46.102(a) Definitions. Titles 45 Public Welfare. 2009 July 14. http://www.hhs.gov/ohrp/humansubjects/regbook2013.pdf. Accessed 20 Mar 2015.
2. California State University: San Marcos. Guidelines for defining systematic investigation and generalizable knowledge. 2015. http://www.csusm.edu/gsr/irb/policy_guidelines/definition.html. Accessed 2 Apr 2015.

 3. Encyclopaedia Britannica: scientific method. 2015. http://www.britannica.com/EBchecked/topic/528929/scientific-method. Accessed 2 Apr 2015.
 4. Haber J. Research question, hypothesis and clinical questions: Chapter 2. 2015. p. 27–55. https://www.us.elsevierhealth.com/media/us/samplechapters/9780323057431/Chapter%2002.pdf. Accessed 2 Apr 2015.
 5. Kumar R. Research methodology: a step-by-step guide for beginners. London: Sage; 2014.
 6. Song JW, Chung KC. Observational studies: cohort and case–control studies. Plast Reconstr Surg. 2010;126(6):2234–42.
 7. Neswiadomy RM. Foundations of nursing research. 5th ed. 2008. wps.prenhall.com/chet_neswiadomy_foundation-5. Accessed 11 Apr 2015.
 8. Glaser BG, Strauss AL. The discovery of grounded theory. Strategies for qualitative research. Piscataway: Transaction Publishers; 2009.
 9. Sbaraini A, Carter SM, Evans RW, Blinkhorn A. How to do a grounded theory study: a worked example of a study of dental practices. BMC Med Res Methodol. 2011;11:128.
10. Koshy E, Koshy V, Waterman H. Action research in healthcare. Chapter 1. 2011. http://www.sagepub.com/upm-data/36584_01_Koshy_et_al_Ch_01.pdf. Accessed 8 May 2015
11. Ressing M, Blettner M, Klug SJ. Systematic literature review and meta-analyses. Part 6 of a series on evaluation of scientific publications. Dtsch Arztebl Int. 2009;106(27):456–63.

Chapter 4
Clinical Trials in Developing Countries: An Overview

Matthys Botha and Michèle Desire Zeier

Abstract The World Health Organization (WHO) defines a clinical trial as "any research study that prospectively assigns human participants or groups of humans to one or more health-related interventions to evaluate the effects on health outcomes".

The clinical trials are needed in order to be able to expand on available cancer treatments, to ensure that a steady pipeline of safe medications reaches the market. Clinical trials may provide a lifeline of newer drugs still in development to patients who have failed previous other treatment options.

A good clinical trial is one that contributes a good volume of data of excellent quality for analysis and achieves this goal according to ethical standards.

The majority of clinical treatment studies in oncology in lesser-developed regions will be phase II or III as most of developing countries may not have the laboratory facilities for complicated studies and may sometimes lack the capacity for management of severe adverse reactions.

Keywords Clinical trials • Phases of trials • Intervention • Newer drugs

M. Botha (✉)
Unit for Gynaecological Oncology, Department of Obstetrics and Gynecology,
Faculty of Health Sciences, Tygerberg Hospital and University of Stellenbosch,
Cape Town, South Africa
e-mail: mhbotha@sun.ac.za

M.D. Zeier
Department of Obstetrics and Gynecology, Faculty of Health Sciences,
University of Stellenbosch, Cape Town, South Africa

© Springer International Publishing Switzerland 2016
D.C. Stefan (ed.), *Cancer Research and Clinical Trials in Developing Countries*, DOI 10.1007/978-3-319-18443-2_4

Introduction

What Is a Clinical Trial?

The World Health Organization (WHO) defines a clinical trial as "any research study that prospectively assigns human participants or groups of humans to one or more health-related interventions to evaluate the effects on health outcomes." Clinical trials might compare new and existing interventions, test new ways to use or combine interventions, or observe how people respond to other factors that might affect their health (such as dietary changes).

In cancer research, as with other chronic diseases, observational studies also have an important purpose. Although not traditionally regarded as clinical trials because no active intervention such as testing new treatment modalities or randomization to treatment arms is performed, these studies usually have minimal investigational aspects outside routine clinical management. For example, in a *prospective* cohort such as a cancer registry, it may involve collection of additional parameters, such as family history, but may also involve some molecular testing or collection of biobanking specimens. *Retrospective* cohorts will only harvest information already collected either from a paper-based patient file or extracting data points from an existing electronic database. As with clinical trials, observational studies must be conducted within the required regulatory and ethics frameworks for conducting research. Observational studies contribute greatly to our understanding of epidemiological trends in chronic diseases and may involve inclusion of thousands of study subjects from numerous contributing sites.

Why Do We Need Clinical Trials?

Simply stated, we need to do research to know what we are doing and why we are doing things as we do now. This starts with having oversight into current epidemiological trends and understanding and monitoring current trends, but also predicting short- to long-term challenges in managing cancer, on a local, national, and international level. We also need research to expand our arsenal of available treatments. Candidate treatments need responsible, dedicated healthcare workers as well as committed patients to ensure that a steady pipeline of safe medications reaches the market. Moreover, research educates both patients and their caregivers about new prevention and treatment modalities and the efficacy and safety of existing ones. Done in an ethical and regulated manner, it can raise the quality of care within and outside of the research setting. Lastly, it may provide a lifeline of newer drugs still in development to patients that have failed previous treatment options.

A Short History of "Evidence-Based Treatments"

Modern, Western medicine claims to be scientifically based. However, much of the underlying assumptions and beliefs are based on historical practice and lack solid scientific proof. "Evidence-based medicine" requires the healthcare provider to evaluate the robustness of the scientific basis of a specific treatment. Modern studies provide data from meta-analyses, systematic reviews, and randomized controlled trials, which may yield strong recommendations and weaker types of data (such as from case–control studies) which yield weak recommendations.

James Lind was born in Edinburgh in 1716. He joined the navy as a helper to the ship's surgeon, but was soon promoted to surgeon. He became aware of the suffering associated with scurvy caused by the vitamin C-deficient diets of the seamen on long ship journeys. Lind was not the first to suggest citrus fruit as a remedy for scurvy, but he was the first to study their effect by a *systematic experiment* in 1747. It was probably one of the first clinical experiments in the history of medicine. He later recommended growing watercress on wet blankets.

An English epidemiologist and statistician, Austin Bradford Hill, studied streptomycin for the treatment of tuberculosis. He used *randomization* and the study is generally accepted as the first randomized clinical trial. In collaboration with Richard Doll, he also described the link between cigarette smoking and lung cancer.

Other well-known pioneers in the field of evidence-based medicine include Archie Cochrane, who was the author of an influential book: *Effectiveness and Efficiency: Random Reflections on Health Services*. His work led to the formation of the Cochrane Collaboration, a non-profit organization with the aim of "making the vast amounts of evidence generated through research useful for informing decisions about health."

Globalization and the Lessons Learned from HIV Research

The HIV epidemic in Southern Africa provides a model from which multinational research can obtain strategies for approaching the conduct of cancer research in the developing world. This is true for both its successes and deficiencies.

One of the most important strengths of international research is collaborative efforts. An example of an international funding model in the field of HIV care is the United States of America President's Emergency Plan for AIDS Relief (PEPFAR), which has contributed funding to development of infrastructure and training of local healthcare workers and worked in partnership with government models. Partly as a result of this funding, South Africa has the largest HIV treatment program in the world. The project has indirectly led to a wealth of epidemiological and interventional data, which have enriched the scientific understanding of HIV epidemiology and management.

Other large funding sources include the Bill and Melinda Gates Foundation, the Global Fund, the Wellcome Trust, and the Joint United Nations Programme on HIV/AIDS (UNAIDS). The lessons learnt from these collaborations include how working with existing structures may lead to success in expanding treatment capabilities with huge benefit to the recipient communities, and these lessons can be extrapolated to smaller-scale intervention studies or drug intervention trials.

Collaborative research in the field of HIV treatment and HIV vaccine research also emphasized the value of having an ethics review system where the protocol and consenting process is defined by Good Clinical Practice and approved by the local Ethics Committees in host countries. Importantly, this process concerns the concept of "Standard of care." Particularly evident at the time when antiretroviral treatment (ART) was not readily available to persons living with HIV infection in South Africa, the dilemma quickly raised itself as what the standard of care should be: that of the sponsor country, where ART programs were up and running, or of the host country, where most patients did not have access to treatment. It quickly became clear that clinical trials had to be constructed in order to provide treatment not usually standard in the host country. Placebo-controlled studies, such as those comparing AZT to placebo in prevention of mother-to-child transmission, would not be ethically acceptable. Also, protocols providing a third ART and comparing it to placebo when added to a nucleoside analogue backbone, did not meet the standard of care in the sponsor country and the nucleoside backbone treatment also had to be funded for South Africa, even if they were not required to do so in the country of origin. Furthermore, post-protocol access to treatment was required and defined as providing continued access in the form of a rollover protocol for as long as the candidate drug was not yet registered for use in the host country, and in the form of continued access programs for as long as the patient could not access treatment post-protocol even after the drug was registered for use. In practical terms, this meant providing ART post-protocol until patients were able to or chose to enrol into the government-sponsored ART program.

It can thus be said that the HIV research community revealed the importance of compassionate research in lesser-developed areas. In cancer trials, many parallel situations exist.

Increased research activities in developing countries may have serious implications for the host country in terms of the risk of exploitation. A range of vulnerabilities depending on localization and size of the specific health burden may include:

- Weak socioeconomic circumstances reflected in constrained healthcare budgets, inadequate resources, and overwhelmed healthcare systems. Examples could include low screening efforts due to cost, long treatment waiting periods, and long and costly patient travel times to treatment centres.
- Inexperienced research facilities, Ethics Review Boards, or investigators, who may be eager to initiate a protocol at their new research site. These problems may be exacerbated by competitive enrolment strategies.
- Disparate distribution of benefit and risk between sponsor and host communities: research subjects in developing countries carry the highest proportion of risk for

researching a new compound to treat a disease that is prevalent in their country, but their community will often never realistically and financially have access to the treatments.

- Study subject access to treatment: after completing participation in a particular study, the subject does not have further access to life-saving medication.
- Cultural and language differences in obtaining informed consent from subjects. Ignoring cultural sensitivities such as community and familial consent may build resistance against research projects in the host country.
- Lack of capacity to move on from pilot studies.

Drivers of Research Agenda in Low-Resource Settings

In spite of these pitfalls in engaging in research in developing countries, the benefits both for host and sponsor mostly outweigh the potential difficulties that may be encountered. Apart from the strengthening of local treatment programs, participants gain access to services not generally available. For the sponsor, conducting a trial in a developing country may be beneficial because larger numbers of patients may be able and willing to enrol due to the added benefit they will receive. Unique study populations, representing different tumour genetics, as well as concomitant disease such as HIV infection, create scientific interest in host population enrolment.

Types of Studies

Observational Studies

Observational studies are sometimes regarded as weak designs with low potential to be scientifically valid. However, in the field of cancer research where current treatments are often unsuccessful or even harmful, observational studies are essential to carefully assess the success (or lack thereof) of accepted treatments. Observational studies help to define the risks associated with treatments and may help to identify links between disease and risk factors. Data for observational studies may be collected retrospectively or prospectively. "It *describes* what is happening rather than *decides* what is happening."

(a) Cohort

A study cohort is a defined study population in which clinical, pathological, molecular, psychosocial, or other aspects are investigated. The study design may be a retrospective or prospective. It describes characteristics of the selected population and tries to find links between parameters that may be clinically useful.

(b) Case–control
   Compares persons with a disease or outcome to a group without the disease or outcome. The aim is to determine the differences or parameters that may explain why cases become affected with the disease.
(c) Biobanking
   A biorepository that stores biological samples for future reference and testing. This is a specialized form of a cohort study. Samples are stored and may later be tested for genetic studies, infectious agents, or disease markers.

Treatment Study

Treatment studies evaluate the impact of an intervention in a study population. Clinical trial interventions include:

- Screening and preventative strategies
- New medication (e.g., chemotherapy, hormones, antibiotics, or targeted drugs), cells, or other biological products
- Surgical, physical (e.g., radiotherapy) treatments and procedures
- Vaccines
- Medical devices (including surgical implants)
- Behavioural and supportive therapies
- Complementary and alternative therapies

Interventions are usually compared to existing and approved treatments. In order to prevent investigator or sponsor bias, these studies are most often performed in a randomized fashion, which means that neither the patient, study team nor pharmaceutical company decide in which treatment (investigative or comparative) arm the patient is placed; the assignment occurs in a statistically random manner. Trial design may involve one of the following levels of randomization:

(a) Non-blinded (Open): both the patient and the investigator know which treatment (investigative or comparative) is given to the patient. This study design may lead to bias on the part of patient or investigator as each may assign efficacy or side-effects according to their experience or prior knowledge with similar treatment modalities.
(b) Single-blind studies: only the researcher knows the assignment of the patient, the patient is not informed. Here the behaviour of the investigator may give subtle clues to the patient. The investigator may also under- or over-report effectiveness and side-effects depending on his or her belief about whether the new intervention is good or not.
(c) Double-blind studies: eliminates patient and investigator bias, as neither knows whether the patient is receiving the active or comparative compound. A study is only truly blinded if the drugs are identical in appearance, colour, and packaging. Unblinding may be necessary in cases of severe or life-threatening toxicity, or when progression of disease has occurred which may require treatment adjustment.

Placebo-controlled is a special type of clinical trial. In a placebo-controlled trial, the comparative drug (the placebo) contains no active ingredient. Placebos are sometimes used in blinded studies. However, these methods are only used if the current standard of care involves no treatment. The study will usually offer an active roll-over for patients who have completed study and had been randomized to the placebo arm, if the drug candidate met the required efficacy and safety standards.

Quality of life assessments provides valuable information either as separate observational studies for patients receiving standard care, or play an additional role in evaluating the effect of a new treatment modality in clinical care, as an extra dimension to drug efficacy and safety outcomes.

Phases of Treatment Studies

Traditionally, treatment studies have been divided into phases to organize the development of new medicines (see Table 4.1).

The majority of clinical treatment studies in oncology in lesser-developed regions will be phase II or III. Developing countries may not have the laboratory facilities for pharmacokinetics (PK) studies and may sometimes lack the capacity for management of severe adverse reactions. The same argument may be made for phase II studies.

Why Cancer Studies Are Different

- Vulnerable population

  Cancer is a feared diagnosis in all cultures. There is often the perception that cancer inevitably leads to death. Treatment options for certain cancer types may be limited and often not successful. This may make patients who are invited to participate in studies vulnerable and open to exploitation. They may feel desperate and scared and agree to participate even when there are risks involved. In the face of the serious nature of disease, risk-benefit will allow often serious (and dangerous) side effects. Ethics committees (usually run by universities or research facilities) aim to prevent exploitation by carefully assessing benefit–risk for the participants. Community advisory boards (CABs) may also help to facilitate communication and understanding between the researcher and the participants. CABs consist of people from the study community who have an understanding of the beliefs, language, and culture, but also the aims of the research. CABs should meet regularly with the researchers at all phases of a study.

- Often pharmaceutical industry-driven

  Development of new drugs can be very expensive and time-consuming. The investment by drug companies may lead to pressure to recruit and complete studies quickly. Systems for continuous ethics review may not be in place in

Table 4.1 Description of phases of treatment studies

Phase	Aim	Explanations
Phase 0	Pharmacodynamics (PD) and pharmacokinetics (PK) in humans	Phase 0 trials are the first in-human trials. Single sub-therapeutic doses of the study drug or treatment are given to a small number of subjects (10–15) to gather preliminary data on the agent's pharmacodynamics (what the drug does to the body) and pharmacokinetics (what the body does to the drugs). For a test drug, the trial documents the absorption, distribution, breakdown and removal (excretion) of the drug, and the drug's interactions within the body, to confirm that these appear to be as expected
Phase 1	Screening for safety	Testing within a small group of people (20–80) to evaluate safety, determine safe dosage ranges, and begin to identify side effects. A drug's side effects could be subtle or long term, or may only happen with a few people, so phase 1 trials are not expected to identify all side effects
Phase 2	Establishing the efficacy of the drug, often against a placebo	Testing with a larger group of people (100–300) to see if it is effective and to further evaluate its safety. The gradual increase in test group size allows less common side effects to be progressively sought
Phase 3	Final confirmation of safety and efficacy	Testing with large groups of people (1000–3000) to confirm its effectiveness, monitor side effects, compare it to commonly used treatments, and collect information that will allow it to be used safely
Phase 4	Surveillance studies after registration	Post-marketing studies delineate additional information, including the treatment's risks, benefits, and optimal use. As such, they are ongoing during the drug's lifetime of active medical use

Modified from Wikipedia

lesser-developed settings, but progress and adverse event reports should be regularly submitted to the sponsor company and the local and partner ethics review boards.

Clinical Trials in Oncology: Getting Started

Deciding to Do Research at Your Practice or Clinic

There are several reasons why physicians choose to participate in research studies. This interest may come from prior research experience, or because they have noticed some interesting clinical trends in their patient population. In oncology, as seen in the HIV epidemic, the interest may be born from the inability to access newer treatment options for their patients, medication may still be in the developmental phase, or may be registered but not available in state-funded programs or reimbursed by private insurance. Importantly, engaging in research purely for study site financial reasons without a real commitment to a culture of research may soon see the site dwindle into an underperforming and uncommitted embarrassment for all involved. Sites that have managed to participate for a decade or more in numerous protocols have a wide understanding of the long-term benefit to their patient population and realize that any financial gain will usually be smaller than expected.

What Is a Good Clinical Trial Site?

A good research site from the research prospective is one that contributes a good volume of data of excellent quality for analysis and achieves this goal according to ethical standards. Although a new site may initially be active in a single study, the patient population is best served by a broadening of protocols to include treatment modalities aimed at recurrence or progression of disease, or quality of life observational studies during and after completion of studies. Expansion of the investigative repertoire may also be achieved by participating in protocols that provide new or evaluate existing preventative interventions, or involve genetic investigation of patients and family members. In addition, collaborative studies can provide expertise not existing at the research site, for example, if biopsy specimens or radiological or molecular investigation are required as part of the protocol. The most effective way to widen the spectrum of disease protocols is by participation in a provincial or national oncology research conglomerate. Researchers enrol study participants to existing studies after becoming active sites and may present their own protocols to the research group. This is especially valuable for rare diseases.

Setting Up the Required Infrastructure

Determining the required infrastructure is one of the two main components in building a clinical trial site. Whether the site will be located within a functioning academic oncology treatment centre or in an existing community-based oncology practice, expansion of at least some aspects will have to be budgeted for even with small and basic research studies. This may include items such as office space, desks, computer, and internet access for research personnel, fridge and freezer space, pharmacy or IP storage areas, a centrifuge to prepare specimens for shipment, or even additional consulting rooms. Office space may be made available by the institution at a rental fee, which should be discussed and fixed prior to constructing an operational budget. This may also apply to telephone and internet costs, study-specific investigations, radiology tests, and procedures such as biopsies and cardiac catheterizations. Developing the required infrastructure may require roughly 30 % of the study budget, but subsequent studies may, of course, utilize the same equipment and therefore reduce budgetary input amounts.

Employing Required Staff

Apart from setting up the infrastructure for a clinical trial site, building a successful research team can be a costly and time-consuming undertaking. The lead researcher should be aware that, although he or she is already directly involved in the diagnostic and treatment aspects of prospective trial participants, he also will have to commit a substantial amount of time on a weekly and daily basis to trial-specific activities. Initially, there might be some time available to accommodate research activities, but as the volume of work related to studies, additional administrative duties and travel time to attend meetings, increases, it may become necessary to hire additional staff to assist with research activities, and even routine clinical and teaching duties.

With incentives such as academic publication, gaining experience with novel diagnostic and treatment modalities, and additional reimbursement, clinical staff such as physicians may be willing to accommodate the additional research duties. This tendency varies, however, from private to academic institutions and can also be influenced by the reimbursement climate in the specific country. Over-burdened doctors are generally not capable of adding more tasks to their workload, and being forced into research may make them unhappy, unwilling, and ineffective members of the research team. It is therefore wise to appoint physicians with research experience, as previous participation usually predicts continued interest.

The bulk of the daily research workload will, however, be carried by the Research or Study Coordinator (SC). Although this person will have many administrative duties, there will be clinical aspects to most trials that may only be done by a qualified nurse, and it may be wise to appoint as the first SC on the team an experienced nurse in Oncology who has served as either study nurse or SC on other studies. As the workload increases, an additional SC may be required, and appointing a person without nursing registration may be a cost-saving measure. Unfortunately, in most countries there is an under-supply of experienced research assistants, resulting in a high turnover of research staff. Complicating the matter is the added cost of permanent appointments—most extra staff are only employed for the duration of the study on temporary contracts. This may prevent potentially gifted staff from leaving the security of permanent salaried employment at larger institutions to join research teams elsewhere even if that means they may be forever locked in a service-only environment. Employing a pharmacist or licensed dispenser is often overlooked during the initial planning phase of a clinical trial site. Investigational products have to be correctly stored, and correct documentation of medication may place an extra burden on the site pharmacist. This is especially true if there is blinding of investigational products involved. Many studies require both blinded and unblinded personnel and this must be factored into resource planning. Bench or fridge space and laminar flow cabinets also have to be planned for in existing pharmacies.

For trial sites located within a private practice environment, retraining or hiring staff for both service and research-related activities may still be relatively uncomplicated, but service staff in many academic institutions are not allowed to perform research-specific tasks, and research staff may not be allowed to assist general staff with their daily duties. This precarious balancing act of cementing a cohesive research-service team should be addressed actively by hospital administrators and joint meetings should be promoted as an integral part of the higher goal, which is to effectively treat patients. In this way, patients have access to newer and affordable treatment, service staff have extra hands to perform some of the duties, and research members are more effective in study recruitment as part of a larger team.

Protocol Development and Budget

The importance of the development of an accurate, detailed study protocol is often underestimated. When the study question is identified, the sponsor and the study site investigator should have regular meetings to discuss the scientific plan, study procedures, and timelines in detail. This usually takes time, but if it is not conducted properly will lead to an unsuccessful and problematic study. Role play to test study procedures will often highlight unexpected logistical difficulties. As part of protocol development, regulatory approval from authorities needs planning and action. Applications to the Medicines Control Council and ethics committees may take many months to complete.

A realistic budget will make success more likely. There are many hidden costs in running a trial. These include application fees to approval authorities, training and certification of staff, setting up of a trial site, and often an institutional fee which is charged on the overall budget. Budgets should make provision for currency fluctuation, inflation, and unexpected cost items. Study financial management is usually the responsibility of the Principal Investigator (PI), but all financial transactions should be carefully documented and discussed regularly with relevant team members. Audited, well-managed finances will ensure the future of a study site and gain the trust of international partners and sponsors. Any suspicion of financial fraud will lead to distrust of all aspects of the trial including the scientific data generated.

Ethics IRB

Research should always be conducted in an ethical manner. This starts with a good clinical conscience. Is the research important? Will it harm, e.g., withhold optimal treatment from any participant? All staff members also have to be continuously and fully trained in the Guidelines to Good Clinical Practice and Certificates, but also adhere to these guidelines. Personnel members also need special training and supervision in the consenting process. Assistance with the consenting process in the form of translation services is crucial. Cultural sensitivity in participation, e.g., where consent from spouses and community members is required, must be taken into consideration. Furthermore, in vulnerable communities, or communities where there is a lack of standard access to treatment, it is recommended that a community forum provide assistance to the research team and ethics review board.

Study site performance should not only be measured from a research perspective. Study subjects are patients first and foremost. Their care must always take precedence over trial participation: never do harm. Over and above the obvious ethics commitments and requirements, the standard of care provided to a patient participating in a research protocol should have positive repercussions to the quality of care to trial participants and non-trial participants by an improved level of expertise and morale among staff and patients.

Recruitment and Retention

Good enrolment rate is of utmost importance. A general awareness among research and service staff, as well as the patients of both the enrolling and planned studies, should be encouraged. This may be tiresome in a busy clinic or practice where every minute in the day counts, but these are necessary practices for good clinical research. Identifying possible candidates before their arrival—at least a day before their scheduled appointments—takes a lot of stress out of the initial consultation, as the paperwork, patient information leaflets, as well as the time scheduled for the appointment can be adjusted. A good electronic patient database can assist with identifying possible candidates, as well as monitoring randomization figures.

A high screening failure rate should be identified early, especially in studies with stringent inclusion and exclusion criteria, and may require additional action to reach enrolment goals. Poor enrolment rates can also be caused by sites initiating a study that is already near closure, and it is wise to investigate the overall, up-to-date total enrolment numbers for all sites involved. Delays caused by Ethics Committees and contractual documents waiting for approval by institutions can also limit screening time. Weekly accrual feedback to staff members and percentage attainment of enrolment goals is an effective tool to motivate performance and allow early corrective action to be taken. Similarly, the retention of subjects should be monitored and high drop-out rates identified and investigated so that corrective actions can take place early.

Data Monitoring

Good quality data is achieved by employing good staff and training them properly for the duties they will be required to perform. This will entail training in GCP, protocol-specific duties by attending the meetings and site-initiation days, as well as additional training such as site-specific data electronic management and monitoring systems. It is the lead investigator's responsibility to ensure that all staff are regularly trained and maintain professional registration in their respective fields.

An important aspect to achieving data quality is the regular monitoring thereof, particularly in identifying weak aspects. This takes the form of internal and external audits. Internal audits are done by staff members such as a dedicated SC, or the PI, but this is mostly not adequate. External audits can be done by a collaborative site, an independent auditor, the Sponsor Auditors, the Research Conglomerate, or even required by the Independent Ethics Committee, the Medicines Control Council, and/or the US Food and Drug Administration (FDA). Audits are valuable in identifying weak data quality and allowing sites to implement timely corrective actions. All sites must have SOPs which may be amended as needed, to omit future shortcomings or protocol violations. These may involve additional training or even additional monitoring procedures with amendments to the study protocol and re-consenting study subjects.

Reporting

A large part of this important duty is usually delegated to a SC. Reporting duties include screening and enrolment logs, dispensing logs, and adverse event logs. Serious adverse event (SAE) logs are also defined by the protocol. Each member of the research team should be vigilant in identifying SAEs, but it is the PI or his/her assigned responsible sub-Investigator who is responsible for the content of the SAE report. The SAE report must be provided to the overseeing authority within 24 h and will have to contain an assessment as to causality, in other words, whether it is related to the study drug. This assessment may be revised at a later stage as more information becomes available.

Ethics Review Boards, funding organizations, and institutional boards require regular progress updates. These will include enrolment numbers and may include regular budget spending updates to Sponsors.

Reporting to peers is also part of research. Presenting research findings educates colleagues within the field and encourages new research. Platforms may be research meetings with oral or poster presentations and publication in peer-reviewed journals. Writing journal articles is time-consuming and difficult, and unfortunately many less-experienced researchers abandon the process. A publication bias unfortunately exists with negative or neutral trial results less likely to be submitted to journals and, if submitted, also less likely to be accepted for publication.

The Future of Clinical Trials

Historically, cancer treatment has been aimed at preventing the proliferation characteristics of tumours. Due to advances in cancer genome research, newer treatments use a precision approach, targeting tumour-specific molecules such as hormone receptors or cancers that harbour a tumour-specific mutation. Clinical trials in future may have to enrol fewer subjects to prove effectiveness, although comparative arms still aimed at traditional targets will, for now, still determine a larger enrolment target. Also, the therapeutic target being investigated may occur only in a very small minority of subjects screened for enrolment, leading to higher screening failure rates and slow accrual to studies. Higher success may be achieved with larger and wider population screening, inclusion of molecular characterization of tumours as routine screening in cancer programs, and widening of clinical trials to include not merely tissue-specific characteristics but also tumour biology. To achieve this, cohorts from provincial and national cancer treatment centres that also serve as clinical trial sites should collaborate in the epidemiological, biological, and treatment evaluation cancer research sites. Training clinical researchers in oncology must be a priority.

Further Reading

Friedman, Furberg, DeMets, editors. Fundamentals of clinical trials. 2010. ISBN 978-1-4419-1586-3
Evidence-based medicine: how to practice and teach it. 4 ed. 2010. Straus ISBN-13: 978–0702031274
South African National Clinical Trials Register. http://www.sanctr.gov.za/

Chapter 5
The Research Protocol

Gilberto Lopes, Gustavo Werutsky, and Patricia Moretto

Abstract The research protocol is defined as the most important document in clinical research which helps the researchers and the scientists to understand the necessity of the study and the way of execution and completion.

The protocol outlines the rationale for the study, its objective, the methodology used, and how the data will be managed and analyzed. It highlights how ethical issues have been considered, and where appropriate, how gender and minority issues are being addressed.

An additional step, after writing the protocol, particularly in large studies with teams of investigators, is to develop what may be called the operations manual for the study.

The full research protocol development takes usually 4 months, but is variable depending on the complexity of the research.

Keywords Protocol • Protocol synopsis • Protocol writing • Template

Introduction

After proper and complete planning of the study, the detailed plan or protocol should be written down. In the development of a clinical trial, the protocol lies in the middle of a linear process (Fig. 5.1). The initial idea for a trial is first translated into a concept, leading to the definition of a protocol, which results in the recruitment of

G. Lopes, M.D., M.B.A. (✉)
Oncoclinicas do Brasil, Rua Maranhão 569/4, São Paulo, SP 01240-001, Brazil
e-mail: glopes.md@gmail.com

G. Werutsky
Latin American Cooperative Oncology Group,
6681, 99A/806 Ipiranga Avenue, Porto Alegre, RS 90619-900, Brazil
e-mail: gustavo.werutsky@lacog.org.br

P. Moretto, M.D., M.Sc.
Oncology, Caxias do Sul University Foundation, Caxias do Sul General Hospital,
Rua Prof. Antônio Vignoli, 255 - Bairro Petrópolis, Caxias do Sul, RS 95070-561, Brazil
e-mail: morettop@hotmail.com

© Springer International Publishing Switzerland 2016
D.C. Stefan (ed.), *Cancer Research and Clinical Trials in Developing Countries*, DOI 10.1007/978-3-319-18443-2_5

Fig. 5.1 The clinical trial process

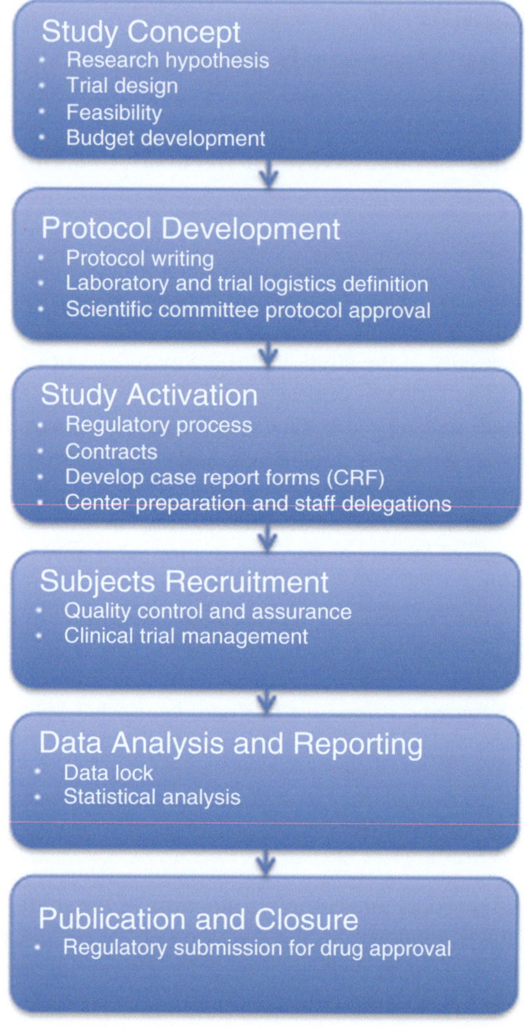

patients (accrual) and finally to the production of evidence for or against the intervention under study. While in the 1970s, a typical protocol was 10 pages long, today's protocols are mostly longer than a hundred pages, evidence of the increasing complexity of human experimentation. Full protocol development usually takes around 4 months. The protocol should outline the rationale for the study, its objective, the methodology used, and how the data will be managed and analyzed. It should highlight how ethical issues have been considered, and where appropriate, how gender and minority issues are being addressed.

The protocol writing process:

- Makes the investigators clarify their thoughts and think about all aspects of the study.
- Is a necessary guide if a team (not a single investigator) is working on the research.

- Is essential if the study involves research on human subjects or experimental animals, in order to get the institution's ethical approval.
- Is an essential component of a research proposal submitted for funding.

During the process of protocol development, investigators can and should try to benefit from the advice of colleagues and experts in refining their plans. But once a protocol has been developed and approved, and the study has started, it should be adhered to strictly and should not be changed. This is particularly important in multi-center studies. Violations of the protocol can discredit the whole study.

An additional step, after writing the protocol, particularly in large studies with teams of investigators, is to develop what may be called the operations manual for the study. This will include detailed instruction to the investigators, e.g., sample collection and handling, to assure a uniform and standardized approach to carrying out the study with good quality control.

Recommended Format for the Research Protocol

This section provides a sample of the format for a research protocol. Investigators should ensure that each of the items included in the format are addressed. It is provided not only to guarantee the highest quality protocol, but also to attend to the ethics review procedure in an efficient and timely manner.

Note that in this template the intervention is a study drug. If the experimental arm is a procedure or a healthcare intervention, the content may be modified as necessary to meet the scientific aims of the study and protocol development.

Title page

	Study title
	type here
Authors	*type here*
Release date	*type here DD-MM-YYYY*

Instructions for Completing the Title Page

Protocol Number

- *Add the protocol (put this number in the page header starting from page 2.*

Study Title

- *Describe the purpose andkey design features of the study.*
- *Use the following elements as appropriate:*

  - *Description of design (e.g., nature of control, blinding, randomization, dosing, and stratification).*
  - *Multicenter or single center.*
  - *Study type (e.g., safety/efficacy/pharmacokinetic/dose-finding/expanded access).*
  - *Brand name, generic name, or investigational drug number.*
  - *Formulation and route of administration.*
  - *Dosage (give in brackets, if applicable).*
  - *Reference therapy (e.g., placebo or active control).*
  - *Subject/patient population and indication.*
  - *Duration of study.*

Authors

- *The authors should be listed in this order as applicable: Study Coordinator (SC), Trial Statistician (TS), Clinical Project Manager (CPM).*

Release Date

- *Release date is the date before or the date on which the document is promoted to "Approved."*

General Instructions

Writing the Protocol

The protocol template contains detailed instructions in each of the sections that will aid the writing of the full protocol. In many cases, specific formats are suggested and menu options and examples are provided. These are intended as guidance, and any given study may need to modify them to some degree, but their use will make protocol writing easier and will lead to consistency in terminology and document structure (Table 5.1).

Table 5.1 Oncology clinical study protocol synopsis

Investigational drug	*Type here_*
Protocol no.	*Type here_* Copy and paste from Title page
Study title	*Type here_* Copy and paste from Title page
Background	Please provide brief background information regarding the study drug including:
	• KEY preclinical/clinical data
	• MAXIMUM three paragraphs
Purpose/rational	Please provide a brief rational for why this study is being conducted; e.g., scientific and/or strategic rational. Also, provide a brief statement on risk/benefits for the patient population
	MAXIMUM one paragraph
Objectives	Precisely worded objectives form the basis for choosing the correct study design, control drugs, assessments, time points for assessment, and methods of analysis in order to generate data that will support the purpose of the study
	Bullet list of the primary objective(s) and only **KEY** secondary objectives
	Primary
	• *Type here_*
	Secondary
	• *Type here_*
Endpoints (efficacy, safety)	List any efficacy or safety endpoints, if applicable
	• *Type here*
Study design	Begin with a **brief** text section, describing the activities of each study phase or period (e.g., screening period, follow-up, survival, treatment period, washout, crossover, etc.)
	State whether an interim analysis is planned and how the information will be used
	State whether a Data Safety and Monitoring Board (DSMB) is planned
	An optional figure outlining the study design may be attached at the end
Population	This section should begin with a **brief** statement describing the patient group for which the study results are generalizable. Additional details should only appear in the inclusion/exclusion (I/E) criteria
Inclusion/exclusion criteria	Bullet list of only **KEY** inclusion and exclusion criteria. This list should be limited to only those criteria that are directly relevant to the trial
	Inclusion
	• *Type here*
	Exclusion
	• *Type here*

(continued)

Table 5.1 (continued)

Investigational and control drugs	The definitions for study drug, study treatment, etc. should agree with the terminologies used in the safety sections of the full protocol
	Study drug refers to any investigational drug(s) or any marketed drug(s) being used for an unapproved indication. Study treatment refers to any combination of study drugs(s), or any combination of study drug(s) and active control(s). Control refers to placebo. Active control refers to any marketed drug used in an approved indication
	For example:
	• Phase III, randomized, Drug A/FOLFOX4 vs. placebo/FOLFOX4
	• Drug A = study drug
	• Placebo = control
	• FOLFOX4 = active control
	• Drug A (or placebo) + FOLFOX4 = study treatment
Dose, regimen, treatment cycle	**Briefly** summarize the dose(s) of study drug/treatment, dosing regimen, and treatment cycle definitions
Supply, preparation, and administration	**Briefly** summarize the following: How supplied; preparation and storage of study treatment; treatment blinding (if applicable); study drug administration; study treatment (i.e., other study drugs) administration; starting dose level for cycle 1 (if applicable); and, number of dose escalation levels (if applicable)
	An optional figure for complicated regimens may be attached at the end
Visit schedule and assessments; efficacy and safety assessment(s)	Briefly summarize key efficacy and safety assessment(s)
Biomarker assessments	**Briefly** summarize biomarker assessments which are testing a particular hypothesis. These should be supported with a secondary objective
Data and Safety Monitoring Board (DMSB)	Yes/no Include purpose, frequency of reviews, internal or external members
Statistical methods and data analysis	**Briefly** summarize the following: Populations for analysis; patient demographics/other baseline characteristics; treatments (study drug, concomitant therapies, compliance); primary objective; secondary objectives; interim analysis; sample-size calculation; and, power for analysis of critical secondary variables

Key dates	FPFV (first patient/ first visit)	LPLV (last patient/ last visit)
	mm/yyyy: *type here_*	mm/yyyy: *type here_*

Number of patients centers and location	Total number of patients: *type here*
	Number of sites: *type here*
	Number of patients per site: *type here*
	Location of sites: *type here*

Background (Limit 2–3 Pages Maximum)

Provide a concise description and overview of:

Disease

- *The condition to be studied and the unmet medical need.*
- *Current treatment options (if available).*

Study Drug

- *Include chemical name, structure (optional), mechanism of action, and also refer to Section for undesirable effects.*

Comparator/Combination Drugs

- *The investigational drug, including mechanism of action, if known, and any previous preclinical, PK, and/or clinical study results that are relevant to an understanding of the protocol (e.g., justification of dose/schedule for study treatment [if not a Phase I study]).*
- *The vision for how the investigational drug will meet the unmet medical need and why this potential benefit outweighs the potential risks associated with study conduct.*
- *If marketed product, please refer to approved product labeling.*

Study Rationale/Purpose

This section should reflect the scientific reason (rationale) for the study and how (purposes) this rationale will be fulfilled. Most studies will have one or more of the following purposes: proof-of-concept; planned for inclusion in initial registration submission, biomarkers, etc.

Objectives

Precisely worded objectives form the basis for choosing the correct study design, control drugs, assessments, time points for assessment, and methods of analysis in order to generate data that will support the purpose of the study.

Primary Objectives

Please note: for all objectives where appropriate, provide end-point in a concise manner with reference to statistical session.

It is recommended that the primary objective meets all or most of these criteria:

- *It must be aligned with the purpose of the study.*
- *Achieving it is considered necessary for the study to have a positive outcome.*

- *It drives the sample-size calculation and any corrections for multiplicity (i.e., the study is powered to achieve this objective).*

A single primary objective is ideal (clear and simple), but two may be necessary for some studies. There may be several secondary objectives.

Secondary Objectives

Often, secondary objectives will be included to evaluate other general properties of the investigational drug (see below), sometimes to evaluate multiple variables, and occasionally to evaluate comparisons with different controls. Other categories of objectives (e.g., tertiary) should be avoided.

Exploratory Objectives (If Necessary)

Some of the biomarker objectives may be purely exploratory in scope. These are hypothesis generating (i.e., discovery-based research) and require separate consent.

Study Design

Provide a brief section, describing the study activities (e.g., screening period, follow-up, survival, treatment period, washout, crossover, etc.).

Provide a single paragraph (for the benefit of the investigators) summarizing the study design (e.g., interim analysis, when the primary and secondary efficacy safety analyses are done, when the study/treatment will be completed, etc.).

When possible, it is highly recommended that a study outline be provided using a schematic or presentation in a table. *This outline should include the following: patient population, stratification, randomization, dosing schema, biomarker assessments, sample-size estimates, etc.*

Population

This section should begin with a general statement describing the characteristics of the patient group for which the study is designed. Additional details should only appear in the I/E criteria.

Inclusion/Exclusion Criteria

Begin with the following statement:

The investigator or his/her designee must ensure that all patients who meet the following inclusion and exclusion criteria are offered enrolment in the study.

Inclusion Criteria

- *Define tumor or other malignancy type (e.g., histologically confirmed colorectal cancer).*
- *Define stage of disease (e.g., first line metastatic).*
- *Define amount of previous treatment allowed.*
- *Define RECIST lesion entry criteria (i.e., measurable, non-measurable).*
- *Others.*

Exclusion Criteria

Please note: be concise and list the criteria in order of:

- *Disease exclusions: Any exclusionary sites of disease (e.g., brain metastases); any particular tumor type/subtypes to be excluded; and, any excluded therapies specific for your study indication, etc.*
- *Conditions that preclude inclusion as laboratorial abnormalities and underline disease states.*
- *Any of concurrent severe and/or uncontrolled medical conditions, which could compromise participation in the study.*
- *Pregnancy and breast-feeding exclusion.*

Treatment

Investigational and Control Drugs

- *Provide clear definitions for study drug, study treatment, etc.*
- ***Study drug*** *refers to:*

  - *Any investigational drug(s).*
  - *Any marketed drug(s) being used for an unapproved indication and/or dose, dose regimen, or dose protocol.*

- ***Study treatment*** *refers to: study drug or combination of study drugs.*
- ***Control****: refers to placebo control or active control (refers to any marketed drug used in an approved indication, dose, and dose regimen).*
- ***Study combination****: a new combination or a combination being used for an unapproved indication.*

Drug Supply, Preparation, and Storage

Treatment Arms

Describe in detail individual arms for trial. Include information about:

- *Route of administration*
- *Amount (e.g., number of tablets taken at a time)*
- *Frequency*

- *Timing*
- *Dosing modifications: dose-reduction criteria for interruption and re-initiation*
- *Duration of treatment*
- *Definition of a treatment cycle*

Other Concomitant Medications

Describe treatment other than study drug, ancillary treatments, or rescue medication that is allowed and not allowed after the start of study drug, including other medications, therapies, exercise, diet, changes in living arrangements, etc.

Study Drug Discontinuation

Define criteria to consider completion of treatment and set a date for last follow-up appointment. For example: If, for any patient, either study treatment or observations are permanently discontinued, the patient will be considered to have completed study treatment. All patients must have evaluations for 28 days after the last dose of study treatment.

Treatment Compliance

Describe methods to ensure and monitor treatment compliance, such as dosing in the presence of the Clinical Research Assistant or by subject diary and drug accountability records.

Patient Numbering

Create a system for patient numbering. This could include a combination of center number (for multi-center trials) and subject number.

End of Treatment

Patients may be withdrawn from the study prematurely for one of the following reasons:

- Adverse event(s)
- Abnormal laboratory value(s)
- Abnormal test procedure result(s)
- Protocol violations
- Withdrawal of consent
- Lost to follow-up

- Administrative problems
- Death
- New cancer therapy *(optional: only to be used for specific requirements)*
- Disease progression

Table 5.2 Visit evaluation schedule (sample)

	Baseline	Cycle 1								Subsequent cycles				End of study treatment	Endpoint follow up[a]
Visit No.	1	2	3	4	5	6	7	8	9	10	11	12	13	14	
Day of cycle	−14 to −1	1	2	3	8	15	16	17	22	1	8	15	28	Last	
Demography/ informed consent	X															
Inclusion/ exclusion criteria	X															
Relevant medical history/ current medical conditions	X															
Diagnosis and extent of cancer	X															
Prior anti-neoplastic therapy	X															
Vital signs	X															
Height	X															
Weight	X															
Physical examination	X															
WHO performance status	X															
Chest X-ray	X															
EKG	X															
Hematology	X															
Coagulation	X															
Biochemistry	X															
Urinalysis	X															

(continued)

Table 5.2 (continued)

	Baseline	Cycle 1										Subsequent cycles					End of study treatment	Endpoint follow up[a]
Serum pregnancy test	X																	
Thyroid function test	X																	
Cardiac enzymes	X																	
Cardiac imaging	X																	
Standard MRI/CT assessment of tumors	X																	
Prior/ concomitant medications	X	Continuous																

The end of the treatment can occur when the duration is completed as per protocol.

Visit Schedule and Assessments

Include descriptions of assessments under the individual subheadings listed below according to the purpose for which the information is collected rather than according to standard definitions (Table 5.2).

Patient Demographics/Other Baseline Characteristics

Describe the data that will be collected on patient characteristics at baseline, including demographic information and other background or medical history (e.g., family history, smoking history, etc.). Also describe other assessments that are done for the purpose of determining eligibility for inclusion in the study (e.g., diagnostic tests) and whether or not the data are to be entered into the database.

Disease Assessment

- Physical examination, weight, height
- Vital signs
- Performance status
- Laboratory evaluations: hematology, coagulation, biochemistry
- Radiological examinations

Treatments

Describe the data that will be collected on the study drug and other therapies used in order to provide information about drug exposure.

Efficacy

- *Use RECIST criteria (if applicable)*
- *Include how and when the tumor data will be collected*

Safety

Use a separate third-level heading for each safety assessment (e.g., adverse events, physical examinations, vital sign measurements, laboratory evaluations).

- **Adverse events**

   An adverse event for the purposes of this protocol is the appearance of (or worsening of any preexisting) undesirable sign(s), symptom(s), or medical condition(s) occurring after signing the informed consent even if the event is not considered to be related to the study drug(s).

- **Pregnancies**

   Example: to ensure patient safety, any pregnancy in a patient on the study drug must be reported to the Sponsor within 24 h of learning of its occurrence.

Safety Monitoring

Adverse Event Monitoring

Subjects will be closely monitored throughout the study for adverse events and will not be discharged from the study until the investigator has determined that adverse events have either completely resolved or are not of clinical significance. If known, the diagnosis of the underlying illness or disorder should be recorded, rather than its individual symptoms. The following information should be captured for all AEs: onset, duration, intensity, seriousness, relationship to study drug, action taken, and treatment required.

Serious Adverse Event Reporting

Insert the following suggested text, choosing from among the options bulleted below:
   To ensure patient safety, every serious adverse event (SAE), **regardless of suspected causality**, occurring

- After the patient has provided informed consent and until 4 weeks after the patient has stopped study treatment/participation.
- After the patient is randomized and until 4 weeks after the patient has stopped study treatment.

Note that all occurrences of overdose must be reported as an SAE. An overdose is defined as the accidental or intentional ingestion or infusion of any dose of a product that is considered both excessive and medically important.

Biomarkers

Describe the rational, methods, and statistics of biomarker studies to be included in this protocol.

Drug Safety Monitoring Board

State whether such a Board will be used. If yes, provide information about the composition of the Board and the scope of its mandate.

Data Collection, Review, and Management

The clinical data management team is in charge of proper Case Report Form (CRF) designing, CRF annotation, database designing, data-entry, data cleaning, discrepancy management, medical coding, data extraction, and database locking. This information should be assessed for quality at regular intervals during a trial.

Site Monitoring

The sponsor or the government usually requires Drug Safety Monitoring Boards (DSMBs). Usually this involves regular visit to the research site, and the clinical research associate (CRA) will provide information (through e-mail, telephone, fax, or regular mail) to the monitoring agency.

Statistical Methods and Data Analysis

Populations for Analysis

Whenever possible, definitions should be developed by project and used for all studies in that project. For populations that require the use of study-specific rules for definition, e.g., per-protocol population, provide those rules or describe when and how they will be decided.

Example for randomized trials:

ITT population: consists of all patients as randomized. Following the intent-to-treat principle, patients will be analyzed according to the treatment they were assigned to at randomization.

Safety population: consists of all randomized patients who received at least one dose of study drug and had at least one post-baseline safety assessment. Patients will be analyzed according to treatment received.

Per-protocol population: consists of all randomized patients who received at least one dose of the randomized study drug and had no major protocol violations. The per-protocol patient population will be identified prior to database lock.
The protocol violations must be specified in the protocol.

Statistical Analysis

Describe how the following endpoints will be analyzed:

- Primary objective
- Secondary objectives
- Safety

Sample-Size Calculation

The sample size should always be sufficient to provide adequate power to address the primary objective of the study. In some cases, the sample size may exceed this amount if it is necessary to provide adequate power to address a specific secondary objective or adequate precision to estimate the size of a treatment effect.

- Statistical hypothesis, model, and method of analysis
    State the null and alternative hypotheses, including the preplanned alpha error for rejecting the null hypothesis and any adjustments to account for multiplicity.

Administrative Procedures

- **Regulatory and ethical compliance**
    For multi-center trials, with participation of EU countries, U.S., and Canada, add:
    This clinical study was designed and shall be implemented and reported in accordance with the protocol, the International Conference on Harmonization of Technical Requirements for Registration of Pharmaceuticals for Human Use (ICH)—Harmonized Tripartite Guidelines for Good Clinical Practice (GCP), with applicable local regulations [including European Directive 2001/20/EC, US Code of Federal Regulations Title 21, and Tri-Council Policy Statement on Ethical Research Involving Humans (TCPS2) for Canada, and with the ethical principles laid down in the Declaration of Helsinki.
    Example: For studies done in developing countries, the ethics rules of each country should be reviewed and followed. Specifically for Brazil, it should be taken into consideration that the Plenary of the National Health Council, on

December 2012, revoked the CNS Resolutions No. 196/96, No. 303/2000, and No. 404/2008, replacing it by CNS Resolution No. 466 (see Appendix), which approves regulatory guidelines and norms to be obeyed as of 13 June 2013. The ethics process has to observe the particularities of the country and consider the wording utilized. For example, in Brazil, "Informed Consent" has been altered to "Process of Informed Consent."

- **Responsibilities of the investigator and IRB/IEC/REB**

  The protocol and the proposed informed consent form must be reviewed and approved by a properly constituted Institutional Review Board/Independent Ethics Committee/Research Ethics Board (IRB/IEC/REB) before the study starts. A signed and dated statement of approval must be given to the sponsor before study initiation. Prior to study commencement, the investigator is required to sign a protocol signature page confirming his/her agreement to conduct the study in accordance with these documents and all of the instructions and procedures found in this protocol, and to give access to all relevant data and records to the sponsor monitors, auditors, IRBs/IECs/REBs, and regulatory authorities as required.

- **Informed consent**

  Eligible patients may only be included in the study after providing written (witnessed, where required by law or regulation), IRB/IEC/REB-approved informed consent, or if incapable of doing so, after such consent has been provided by a legally acceptable representative. Informed consent must be obtained before conducting any study-specific procedures (i.e., all the procedures described in the protocol).

Case Report Forms

An investigator is required to prepare and maintain adequate and accurate case histories designed to record all observations and other data pertinent to the investigation on each individual treated or entered as a control in the investigation. Data reported on the CRF that are derived from source documents must be consistent with the source documents or the discrepancies must be explained.

Publications Policy

It is very important to describe who has ownership of the data collected during the study, of publications or abstracts arising from study results, and of information obtained based on new data analyses. For the purposes of filing a patent application, the sponsor may request a delay in publication, and this should be previously specified.

Barriers to Research in Developing Countries and Possible Steps to Overcome Them

The rise in the number of cancer cases, 14 million new cancer cases globally every year, with the majority of cases occurring in developing countries [1], has a great impact in those countries and must be addressed. Additionally, treatment options are both limited and expensive, and trial participation is an opportunity for better cancer care.

There are four key components to cancer control and, therefore, areas in need of research: prevention, early detection, diagnosis and treatment, and palliation, as stated by WHO [2]. In each of these areas, developing countries face major challenges, not only in dealing with the ongoing problems, but also with research opportunities.

The International Agency for Research on Cancer (IARC) uses the term "developing country" for less-developed regions such as: all regions of Africa, Asia (excluding Japan), Latin America and the Caribbean, Melanesia, Micronesia, and Polynesia [1].

In order to overcome barriers to doing research, and so that the results will have a chance to impact on local problems, some points have to be taken into consideration:

Choose a Relevant Topic to Your Community

Make sure that the many pressing problems in developing countries are being addressed, so local patients are able to see direct benefits. The research question has to be relevant for the population where it is tested. This is an ethics question, as well as a question that will improve accrual.

There is a broad consensus that efforts and scarce resources in developing countries should focus first and foremost on prevention and awareness rising, and secondly on early detection, treatment, and research. However, this should not prevent the progress and improvement of research capabilities in these countries.

Will the Protocol Be Feasible?

If the issue being looked at is technology, it should be noted that most health equipment used in developing nations is manufactured in the first world. Sometimes the equipment does not work on arrival, with lack of parts or trained technicians to fix it or do maintenance. Technical, social, cultural, and economic factors must be considered when looking at new technologies for these countries.

Researchers should also remember that in some countries there is limited access to radiotherapy, so research questions involving concurrent or sequential treatments may not be the best research option.

According to the International Atomic Energy Agency (IAEA) [3], although the developing world constitutes 85 % of the world's population, it only has 2200 radiation therapy machines compared with the 4500 in the developed world. Those developing countries that have access to radiotherapy face considerable financial investment constrains and for up to 5 years are required to provide the necessary training, equipment set-up and maintenance, protocols, and quality control. Therefore, even if budget is not a concern for a specific study, creating a Radiotherapy Service for research purposes in a developing country would take a lot of planning, resources, and time.

In order to do the scans as planned in a protocol, radiologists with RECIST knowledge and time to do proper comparative reports are also needed and are not always available. Even with a central review, the delay in getting the images as planned could result in wrong clinical decisions and protocol violations.

The same applies to health workers, where it is sometimes necessary to train locals and adapt to the capabilities of the country. Obviously, if feasible, the improvement in capabilities would be welcome, as in addition to the research they could offer new treatments to patients and open the way for further research.

Funding and Economic Incentives

The challenges are many and substantial such as insufficient political priority and funding among donor agencies and governments of developing countries that have many competing priorities.

However, the local investigator must be familiarized with potential local and international sources: universities, government incentives, international for-profit initiatives, and creative not-for-profit partnerships.

Involvement in research with pharmaceutical companies, which can be lucrative to the institutions where it is done, is an obvious way to start, but usually some capabilities must already be in place to attract this kind of research. A pressing challenge is getting industry partners to invest in the clinical development of drugs that offer limited commercial opportunities. Despite the fact that the cost to approve drugs is lower in developing countries, it is still high and is a problem that universities and public institutions cannot overcome alone.

Intellectual Property

Partnership with industry may be necessary to develop early research in universities, and intellectual property licensing should be viewed as a requirement to attract industry partners. However, researchers must pay attention to patent systems before concluding agreements with pharmaceutical companies (who want a patent system that will protect their investments for as long as possible) and be careful, clearly stating on contracts who has ownership of the data collected, of publications or abstracts arising from study results, and of information obtained based on new data analyses.

Encouragement and Structure

In some developing countries, in addition to other research barriers, such as lack of diagnostic, treatment, and monitoring capacity, there is lack of academic staff (oncology and hematology expertise, specialized cancer nurses, pharmacists), qualified monitors, lack of encouragement to conduct and publish research, as well as lack of a research publishing infrastructure. Training personnel abroad, in other research centers, or in-house training before starting a project may be needed.

Planning and Accrual

Researchers may have problems with proper calculation for accrual, as most cancer registries in low- and middle-income countries have shortcomings and screening programs are largely absent. This can lead to erroneous assumptions regarding the relative frequencies of the varying levels of different cancers based on global trends, which can be misleading. These issues are major challenges for the future, but setting up an institutional cancer registry could be a good start in research planning.

In order to properly choose the study population, the researcher should take into consideration the contrasts in patient's disease profiles: most cancer patients in developing countries have advanced or incurable cancers at the time their initial presentation, a different profile from that seen in developed countries. The prevalence and incidence can be also markedly different in comparison to developed countries for each disease site.

Developed countries often have relatively high rates of lung, colorectal, breast, and prostate cancer because of the earlier onset of the tobacco epidemic, the earlier exposure to occupational carcinogens, and the Western diet and lifestyle. In contrast, up to a fourth of cancers in developing countries are associated with chronic infections. Liver cancer is often causally associated with infection by the hepatitis B virus (HBV), cervical cancer is associated with infection by certain types of human papillomavirus (HPV), and stomach cancer is associated with *Helicobacter pylori* infection.

Weak referral systems can also make the accrual slow. This should be anticipated and should encourage creative solutions to strengthen it by the researchers. In some countries there are few cancer services. This can be helpful in the sense that it aggregates most of the cases in a few centers. However, if the health system is a mix of public and private, this dilutes the number of cases, increasing the numbers of institutions necessary for the accrual, and increasing the budget.

Issues During the Trial and for Follow-Up

There is sometimes a lack of awareness of the signs and symptoms of cancer and side effects from treatments, a lack of money to travel to a hospital, which could result in sub-notification of important events or delays in the notification and treatment of important side effects.

As health systems in developing countries are not set up for chronic disease management, chronic diseases such as cancer are often lost to follow-up. Therefore, organizing proper follow-up for patients enrolled in the trials could be a problem.

Need for Palliative Care Research

In some developing countries, there is lack of trained personnel to administer palliative care or pain killers such as morphine. This is particularly startling given that approximately 70 % of the patients seen at these hospitals are at such an advanced stage of cancer upon arrival that they are beyond cure and palliative care and pain management is the only benefit they can still receive. Studies in the palliative setting, which should be relatively easy to accrue, could have a major impact in the quality of life of patients and in the training of local health workers.

Ethics Barriers

The ethics principles in clinical research were established in order to avoid previous abuses/misconducts, such as the Tuskegee Study of Untreated Syphilis (TSUS).

Based on the influential codes of ethics and regulations that guide ethical clinical research (Nuremberg Code[1]; Declaration of Helsinki[1], Belmont Report[1], CIOMS[1], U.S. Common Rule[1]), seven main principles have been described as guiding the conduct of ethical research[1]: social and clinical value; scientific validity; fair subject selection; favorable risk-benefit ratio; independent review; informed consent; and respect for potential and enrolled subjects.

The trial should follow the ethics rules from the country where it was originally written and in the other countries where the research will be developed. Some areas of ethics controversy in developing countries are: the standard of care to be used (as the local standard of care could mean no treatment or less than the "worldwide best") and the quality of informed consent (due to lack of knowledge, language/ cultural barriers, high workload, and time constraints). The discussion about valid science, social benefits, and favorable risk:benefit ratio to justify less than the worldwide best care has to take place early on in the protocol design to avoid an unethical and/or unfeasible trial. Efforts should be taken to improve the quality of informed consent, such as researchers training and observance to the GCP.

Not all the population in developing countries is vulnerable, but a great deal of them is at increased risk of exploitation due to poverty, limited healthcare services, illiteracy, cultural and linguistic differences, and limited understanding of the nature

---

[1]Conselho Nacional de Saúde (Brasil). Resolução n o 466, de 12 de dezembro de 2012. Brasília, 2012 [citado 2014 Mar 11]. http://www.conselho.saude.gov.br/web_comissoes/conep/index.html. Assessed November 2014.

of scientific research. To make things worse, regulatory infrastructures, which could minimize this risk, may lack effectiveness or be nonexistent. As suggested by Emanuael et al. [4], "collaborative partnerships between researchers and sponsors in developed countries and researchers, policy makers, and communities in developing countries help to minimize the possibility of exploitation by ensuring that a developing country determines for itself whether the research is acceptable and responsive to the community's health problems."

Lastly, the many differences between developed and developing countries, in addition to the various sociocultural groups existing in a country, must be taken into consideration during the research protocol conception and execution. Specifically, issues to keep private information confidential, to find the person responsible for giving consent, and how best to explain the clinical trial purpose, benefits, risks, and involved procedures could arise due to local peculiarities.

References

1. IARC cancer statistics. http://globocan.iarc.fr/. Assessed November 2014. OR http://www.iarc.fr/en/media-centre/pr/2014/pdfs/pr224_E.pdf. Assessed Nov 2014.
2. WHO. Cancer fact sheet. Geneva: WHO; 2014. Accessed Nov 2014.
3. IAEA. A silent crisis: cancer treatment in developing countries. Vienna: Division of Public Information, IAEA; 2003.
4. Emanuel EJ, Wendler D, Killen J, Grady C. What makes clinical research in developing countries ethical? The benchmarks of ethical research. J Infect Dis. 2004;189(5):930–7. Epub 2004 Feb 17.

Chapter 6
Ethics of Conducting Cancer Research in Developing Countries

Jean Marie Kabongo Mpolesha, Mala Ali Mapatano, Ahmed Elzawawy, and Zandile June-Rose Mchiza

Abstract In low- and middle-income countries, the number of externally sponsored clinical cancer studies has doubled in recent years. Cancer research is also on the rise in Africa with the continent hosting over 40 % of clinical trial study sites located outside developed countries.

There is need for the research in the developing world to be accompanied by an understanding of the principles of responsible research conduct to ensure that advances in healthcare are equitably shared and achieved without exploitation.

This chapter outlines ethical issues in developing countries, with a particular focus on the challenges experienced by the *research ethics review committees* (RERCs) in these countries.

Keywords Ethics regulations • Autonomy • Beneficence and non-maleficence • Justice • Plagiarism • Forgery and the falsification of data • Informed consent • Confidentiality

J.M.K. Mpolesha, M.D., Ph.D. (✉)
Department of Pathology, University Hospital,
Zaba, 64 bis, Mbanza-Lemba, Kinshasa, Democratic Republic of Congo
e-mail: mpolkabongo@yahoo.fr

M.A. Mapatano, M.D., M.P.H., Ph.D.
Kinshasa School of Public Health, Department of Nutrition, Room 114, P.O. Box 11850, Kinshasa 1, Democratic Republic of Congo

A. Elzawawy, M.D. Ph.D. Med.
Department of Clinical Oncology and Nuclear Medicine, Faculty of Medicine, Suez Canal University, Ismailia and Alsoliman Clinical and Radiation Oncology Centre, Port Said, Egypt

Z.J-R. Mchiza, Ph.D. Med.
Population Health, Health Systems and Innovation, Human Sciences Research Council of South Africa, 12th Floor Plein Park Building, 69-83 Plein Street, Cape Town 8001, South Africa
e-mail: zmchiza@hsrc.ac.za

© Springer International Publishing Switzerland 2016
D.C. Stefan (ed.), *Cancer Research and Clinical Trials in Developing Countries*, DOI 10.1007/978-3-319-18443-2_6

Introduction: The Cancer Problem in Developing Countries

There is dearth of data regarding ethics and cancer research in developing countries, even though numerous studies have shown that cancer prevalence has risen unevenly across regions and populations over the past two decades [1]. A few of the available studies on ethics suggest that unethical cancer research conduct is rife in developing countries, therefore ethics regulations may need to be adapted to meet current and future scientific advances. Cancer research in developing countries needs to comply with laws and other requirements for research involving human subjects.

However, it is important to highlight that in developing countries researchers conducting studies involving human participants can face significant ethical challenges. While such ethical challenges are common in all health research, cancer research may have some peculiarities of its own, given that cancer research participants may be vulnerable to anxiety and depression [2] or are living with an altered quality of life [3]. In addition, investigators habitually use expensive, time-consuming, labor-intensive, and complex medical procedures.

More importantly, the capacity to develop and use scientific evidence is not equally distributed across continents. Low- to medium-income countries (LMICs) lag behind wealthier nations particularly in terms of the ability of research sites to lead broad, independent clinical research programs [4, 5]. One of the reasons for the setback in most of these countries is the allocation of a meager fraction of the national budget to health research [6]. The limited capacity to conduct health research is itself a public health concern. Public health focuses on creating conditions that enable populations to achieve their highest level of health through prevention of disease and strategies for stopping progression or transmission [7]. Without adequate health research, public health interventions and programs lack a solid evidence base, and not only may they fail to improve health, they may even expose populations to risk.

In this regard, there is urgency to put the cancer and other chronic diseases research agenda at the forefront of the political agenda. National governments need to activate funding for Regulatory and Research Ethics Review Bodies that will monitor and control the conduct of cancer research. Moreover, there is a need to improve the quality of cancer research in developing countries by enhancing international cooperation and exchange of scientific information so as to motivate private international funders to support developing countries research activities [8, 9].

The World Health Organization [10] and the GLOBOCAN [1], the new version of the IARC's online database, highlight that incidence and mortality data quality in most developing countries are not of a high enough standard, despite the increasing cancer burden which estimates that approximately 72 % of cancer deaths occur in these countries. Moreover, when viewing available incidence and mortality data and using the estimated and modelled data recorded in the GLOBOCAN [1] website, it is shown more than half (57 %, $n = 8$ million) of new cancer cases and nearly two thirds of related deaths (65 %, $n = 5.3$ million) occur in the less-developed regions of the planet [1]. A concerning observation in the available cancer data is that, although cancer incidence in developing countries, such as in Eastern Africa, is still lower when compared to new cases per 100,000 women diagnosed annually in Western countries, mortality rates are nearly identical (about 15 per 100,000) in these countries. This seems to suggest that women in Eastern Africa are diagnosed at later stages and therefore have worse survival [1]. It is typical that in developing countries, access to screening and cancer treatment tends to be limited to the most affluent populations, most specifically to the insured minority [11]. Those patients regarded as poor only receive "affordable" or "available" rather than "optimal" treatment. Moreover, those with little chance of benefitting from cancer treatment in accredited health centers, or without financial support, resort to traditional and spiritual healers or are sent home to die, mostly without even the comfort of palliative care [11]. Developing countries are also undergoing rapid societal, economic, and nutrition transition, hence the escalated cancer rates [12].

Putting cancer surveillance and prevention strategies high on the political agenda in developing countries may be the best way to halt this epidemic. Doing so will fast-track cancer research (more specifically, clinical, laboratory, and public health research) in these countries. Furthermore, efforts to implement primary prevention of cancer in developing countries will likely involve detecting those at risk earlier (through surveillance and screening), providing treatment (of optimum quality) in the early stages of the diseases, as well as providing prevention strategies to those at risk of developing the disease.

This is by no means an easy task, since many of the developing countries are already overburdened, trying to fast-track research directed at timely diagnosing and providing adequate care and monitoring for other chronic communicable and non-communicable diseases that have also escalated as the result of urbanization and globalization. Moreover, the rising prices of medicines and vaccines are putting cancer control beyond the reach of many governments in developing countries.

Methodology

In order to write this chapter, we conducted a literature review on ethics and cancer research in different LMICs (see Box 6.1). The review helped in outlining ethical issues with regard to health research conduct in developing countries, with close consideration of the Belmont Report [13]: autonomy, beneficence, and justice. In addition, we considered some elements of research integrity that are important to cancer research investigators, namely the avoidance of plagiarism, forgery, and the falsification of data.

Our review gave us an overview of the situation in cancer research in developing countries and the ethical challenges that arise when conducting this research (see Table 6.1). This information helped in the development of a guide for conducting cancer research in developing countries. As such, the next sections will focus on two distinct topics namely the: (1) current structure and function of research ethics review committees in developing countries; and (2) research conduct in developing

> **Box 6.1: Search Strategy**
>
> We accessed peer-reviewed articles, reports, reviews, and chapters that presented data on ethics and cancer research in developing countries between January 1990 and January 2015 from Pubmed/Medline, Google Scholar, ScienceDirect, Medical Complete and Cochrane using the key words "ethics" "cancer research" and "developing countries." For comparison purposes, data on cancer research for different developing countries from the World Health Organization: International Agency for Research on Cancer (IARC) 2014, as well as GLOBOCAN 2012, the new version of the IARC online database, were also used. The timeframe of 1990 to January 2015 was selected because it was reasonable enough to show publications related to ethics and cancer research in developing countries, since this research topic is fairly new in these countries. All publications falling within this time period that had available and accessible abstracts and full text were included.

countries. These topics helped in the formulation of the developing country-specific practical guide (Table 6.1) to be followed by cancer researchers when conducting research in developing countries.

Before we outline the ethics areas of concern in conducting research in developing countries, we would like to outline the situation of research ethics review committees (RERCs) in developing countries:

The Current Structure and Function of Research Ethics Review Committees in Developing Countries

The RERCs in developing countries do not seem to be representative of the research activities taking place in these countries. According to Bartlett [14], there are fewer ($N=190$) and ($N=85$) institutional review boards (IRBs) that represent 20 Latin American and 26 African countries, respectively, when compared to 324 IRBs representing only two North American countries. In fact, Kass et al.'s. [15] case study on RERCs in Africa showed that 36 % of IRB member countries had no RERCs [15]. Rivera and Ezcurra [16], on the other hand, showed that only 25 RERCs are particularly active in the implementation of collaborative research in 26 Latin American countries. This therefore raises the concern that developing countries may be overburdened with the workload of making sure that the research done in these countries conforms to international ethics standards. Indeed, when Kass et al. [15] and Rivera and Ezcurra [16] conducted their analysis of RERCs in these two countries, they found that staff in most of the RERCs were overburdened with work and had multiple responsibilities, such that they were responsible not only for

Table 6.1 A developing country-specific practical guide to cancer research

What you need to know	Barriers to conducting cancer research in LIMICs	Possible solutions to overcome these barriers
Competency in ethics in cancer research and Good clinical practice (GCP) training is mandatory	• Budget constraints make it difficult to attract experts in research ethics • Limited capacity development or no training at all is received by the few RERCs representatives • Return of results that have not been clinically validated; problems associated with researchers who do not have a clinical practice background [14–16, 29]	• Teaching ethics to undergraduate and postgraduate medical students • Reverting back to the fundamentals of the medical profession; teaching medical ethics and enforcement of "medical neutrality" by embarking some grade of "medical immunity" on the basis of the oath is necessary for the ethical conduct of research • Making GCP training a prerequisite to all cancer researchers [8, 38]
The research protocol must be sound and have value—i.e., it must bring new knowledge that will improve the health status of the nation	• Cancer clinical trials (chemotherapy and vaccines, in particular) are difficult to implement and maintain in developing countries, thereby raising concerns and debates about the effectiveness and the long-term side-effects of these medicines and vaccines • Patients from developing countries are sometimes included in clinical trials evaluating the role of treatments that are unlikely to be made available to them after the trial because of prohibitive costs [39–41]	• More research needs to be implemented to show the long-term effectiveness of chemotherapy and vaccines • Upfront arrangements ensuring post-trial access to proven interventions in developing countries is probably a better alternative than exclusion from the research • Under no circumstances should a study ever be permitted to satisfy regulatory requirements for licensing approval in the "developed" world if there is reliable evidence that *any* of the human subjects entered into that trial were not treated with adequate safeguards, or that ethically mandated informed consent procedures designed to respect the autonomy and dignity of all people were not employed [34, 41]

(continued)

Table 6.1 (continued)

What you need to know	Barriers to conducting cancer research in LIMICs	Possible solutions to overcome these barriers
Research and new drugs or treatment have to pass review before implementation	• Developing countries' RERCs are not necessarily representative of the research activities taking place in developing countries. As such they seem to be overburdened [14–16]	• National governments need to put the cancer research agenda at the forefront of the political agenda • National governments need to activate funding for Regulatory and Research Ethics Review Bodies that will monitor and control the conduct of cancer research • There is a need to enhance international cooperation and exchanges of scientific information to motivate private international funders to support research activities in developing countries [8, 9, 34]
Reputable sources of funding should be attracted as potential sponsors or funders for cancer research	• Few independent funders fund research conducted in LIMICs	• There is a need to enhance international cooperation and exchanges of scientific information so as to motivate private international funders, philanthropists, international agencies with no hidden agendas, and non-governmental organizations to support developing countries' research activities
	• Governments in LIMICs have limited funds directed to cancer research due to the focus on strategies to alleviate poverty with major health expenditure still directed at combating infectious diseases	• Promote opportunities for collaborative research and training in developing countries
	• Funders of cancer research are mostly non-reputable sources (pharmaceutical companies, in particular, that may have hidden agendas) [15]	• Governments need to prioritize cancer research [8, 9]
Fair subject selection procedures need to be followed at all times	• Community-based research frequently occurs in the context of multiple and intersecting social, political, and economic problems. This can result in uneven and unethical selection of participants [15, 42]	• No population of people can be included or excluded from research or unfairly burdened unless there is an overwhelming reason to do so [21]

A comprehensive informed consent document that is not too long and is comprehensible to participants is a prerequisite for all human subjects and their families	• Many of the informed consent forms (ICFs) for industry-sponsored trials are incomprehensible to many participants. The way in which HPV vaccines are often promoted to women indicates that such disclosure is not always given from the basis of the best available knowledge	• Human subjects must voluntarily consent to research and be allowed to discontinue participation at any time
	• Ethical issues arise regarding dosage, logistics, vaccine storage, HPV vaccine acceptability, and cost-effectiveness of vaccine coverage in low-resourced countries	• Research involving human subjects must be valuable to society and provide a reasonably expected benefit proportionate to the burden requested of the research participant
	• Including vulnerable subjects [21, 43, 44]	• Research participants must be protected and safe. No research is more valuable than human well-being and human life
		• Researchers must avoid harm, injury, and death of research subjects and discontinue research that might cause harm, injury, or death
		• Research must be conducted by responsible and qualified researchers [21]

(continued)

Table 6.1 (continued)

What you need to know	Barriers to conducting cancer research in LIMICs	Possible solutions to overcome these barriers
Data need to be kept confidential and safe	• Reviewing archived health information of civilians attending government-controlled health facilities or information on the deceased kept at the government-controlled mortuaries without proper consent from patients or relatives (family)	Prerequisites to storage and re-use of data
	• In addition there are also operational issues which include the disposing and sharing biological specimens with other international collaborators without the participants' consent, as well as storage of specimens beyond the stipulated and agreed time frame and the communication of data with other collaborators who are not part of the original study	• Gaining consent to archive data at the time of fieldwork
	• Data mismanagement [28, 29]	• Anonymization of data is a traditional option which includes removing identifying information and disguising real names
		• Restricted access (controlled by the host repository) where access to data can be restricted to bona fide researchers for genuine research purposes
		• Restricted access (controlled by the depositor)
		• User undertakings (controlled by the host repository) which require users to sign a document setting out terms and conditions of re-use
		• Re-contacting participants. It is possible for principal investigators to go back to research participants to obtain consent for deposit of their data in a public archive [28]
Avoidance of plagiarism, forgery, and falsification of data	• Lack of competency in English, receiving research funding from non-reputable sources, and hunger for outputs due to the pressure to maintain research careers have been given as the reasons why scientists fabricate and manipulate results or conduct plagiarism in developing countries [36, 37]	All cancer researchers

reviewing the research conducted by the centers with which they are directly affiliated, but also for research conducted by other associated centers.

Another issue of concern is the professional diversity of the representatives within RERCs in developing countries. For instance, Rivera and Ezcurra's Latin American [16] study found that of the 191 RERCs members identified, the majority (63 %) were physicians followed by basic or social scientists, lawyers, nurses, or community representatives (≤11 %). This lack of diversity has also been highlighted in RERC representatives in Africa. Of the 31 RERC representatives identified in a case study by Kass et al. [15], most were clinicians, with fewer social scientists, economists, nutritionists, pharmacists, statisticians, lawyers, and lay persons or non-scientists. This is cause for concern, as it means that the rights and welfare of human subjects might not be optimally protected during the research review processes in developing countries. An essential requirement of the Code of Federal Regulations for the protection of human research subjects, Title 45 Part 46 (45 CFR 46) [17], suggests that in addition to scientists and other professionals, institutional review boards (IRBs) must have members that are diverse in race, gender, and cultural backgrounds for them to be sensitive to issues such as community attitudes [17].

The majority of RERCs in developing countries grapple with *budget constraints*. This means it is difficult to attract representatives who are experts in research ethics, resulting in research protocols reviewed by less-specialized representatives. Moreover, lack of administrative support and the other resources within the RERC institutions are constantly reported. This means that representatives who already struggle to cope with their workload are conducting their own admin work. This contributes to the burden of work and lack of sufficient time to review in due time. To cope with these constraints, some RERCs may compromise their integrity and expedite or receive funds from non-reputable sources, bypassing the laws of ethics in research [15].

Another issue highlighted by reviewers of RERCs operation in developing countries is the lower frequency of meetings within committees. Substantiated evidence [14–16] suggests that the majority of RERCs in developing countries, Africa and Latin America, specifically meet either irregularly (three or less times) within a 12-month period. When they do meet, not all of these RERCs produce minutes. Moreover, less than 50 % of these RERCs have established formal operational procedures.

Another major concerning challenge for conducting research in low-resourced communities in developing countries is *conflict of interest*. First, we would like to highlight the political interference and culture of corruption that is seen by researchers as compromising the integrity of the RERCs [15]. There is also some concern regarding the expedited review of rejected research proposals in developing countries. This process does not require a full committee review meeting; sometimes it includes top management individuals who might not be research ethics experts. Other potential conflicts of interest raised in developing countries are: (1) favor regarding reviewing a protocol submitted by a departmental colleague; (2) unease in voicing objections when fellow members' protocols were reviewed, fearing being labelled unfriendly; and (3) institutions and community members being unwilling to reject protocols understood to bring employment. These findings are not restricted to developing countries, but have a considerable effect on the ethics procedures.

The *competence and expertise of staff* in many RERCs leaves a lot to be desired. This issue has been a continuous concern to many reviews conducted in developing countries [14–16]. We have already mentioned that budget constraints make it difficult to attract representatives who are experts in research ethics. Moreover, limited capacity development or no training at all is received by those few representatives that the RERCs manage to retain. For instance, in Kass et al. [15] only 6 of the 12 representatives who took part in the research had received ethics training which was externally funded. Moreover, only one of the RERCs investigated offered Good Clinical Practice courses semi-annually.

This evidence outlines the challenges experienced by RERCs in developing countries. Budget constraints are shown to drive these challenges. This is cause for concern since RERCs need to function optimally to regulate research in developing countries and promote good clinical practice. This has consequences for the conduct of research in developing countries. The next section focuses specifically on the ethical challenges in conducting cancer research in developing countries.

Research Conduct in Developing Countries: Ethical Issues in Public Health and Clinical Research

The ethical issues concerning research with human subjects involve topics ranging from voluntary participation, confidentiality in research to fair selection and justice. Some researchers choose to be selective in including participants [18] and in this way breaching ethics guidelines. Sometimes, researchers prefer working with individuals from disadvantaged groups since they are easily manipulated to take part in research [19]. In cancer research, these issues tend to be more magnified, as these individuals may already be vulnerable to anxiety and depression due to their increased cancer risk, or are already living with an altered quality of life due to cancer.

Indeed, Verástegui et al. [19] have shown that the Western drug companies increasingly view Latin America as a good place for clinical research trials, because of the large populations, modern medical facilities, and because large numbers of the population fall into the low-income bracket. When she tried to gain insight into the state of the informed consent signed by participants in the clinical trials endorsed by these Western drug companies, Verástegui [19] found that ethics in cancer trials undertaken in a major cancer center in Mexico (a developing country) may have been breached. The validity of the informed consent forms signed by participants with advanced stage cancer was questionable as they were lengthy and required complex information, with the majority of participants in these trials characterized as poor, with limited or no education [19]. Moreover, Ali et al. [20] highlighted concerns about the ethics of conducting clinical trials in India due to inadequate regulatory oversight and the potential risks of inadequate informed consent, giving incentives and exploitation of participants, particularly the poor and illiterate.

This is a cause for concern in that researchers have the obligation to be sensitive to the special needs of vulnerable individuals. Special justification is required to invite vulnerable persons to participate in research. However, we should appreciate that "no population of people can be excluded from research or unfairly burdened unless there is an overwhelming reason to do so" (*A guide to research ethics. University of Minnesota Center for Bioethics. 2003*) [21].

Moreover, the Council for International Organizations of Medical Sciences (CIOMS) [22] requires that the rights and welfare of these individuals be protected. This may involve limits to the amount of risk allowed in the research underway, consent provided by proxy or surrogate decision making that utilizes the best interest standard, consent monitoring as well as the issue of remuneration/undue influence to participate in the research [23].

Another ethical issue in developing countries comes with research directed at disease surveillance or health-indicator identification in countries. This kind of research is done via community surveys that are aimed at providing better understanding of the health status of civilians. In cancer research, these often include screening procedures that are both noninvasive and invasive. Because of the nature of cancer research, low response rates are often a big challenge. Indeed, Sadetzki et al. [24] have shown that in developing countries such as India or developed countries such as New Zealand, researchers are facing challenges in the recruitment of participants for cancer studies despite the increased risk and larger number of expected cases in these countries.

Informed consent has two main aims. The first is to respect and promote participants' autonomy; and the second is to protect them from potential harm. However, in some developing countries researchers tend to overlook the importance of giving enough information and miss obtaining consent from participants, as they view the survey as mandatory (i.e., it is endorsed by the government). If they do give some form of information, they give less comprehensive information and sometimes don't give the participants time to digest the information so as to give informed consent. For those community participants regarded as illiterate, the researchers tend not to even bother explaining the details of the procedures and justify the issue of no consent by branding the participants as illiterate. The situations described above are fortunately not applicable to all developing countries but are still encountered in some.

Mudur [25] showed that investigators from the Institute of Cytology and Preventive Oncology in New Delhi breached ethics by not obtaining written consent from their participants in a study of rates of progression of uterine cervical dysplasias to malignancy, stating that most of the women in the study were illiterate and that written consent was not mandatory when the study was launched. However, the ethics experts investigating this allegation rejected the argument that written consent was considered unnecessary because the women were illiterate. They highlighted that "Illiteracy is not stupidity," and also cited the sections from the Belmont Report that: "The ethical process demands evidence that the participants must be allowed to volunteer after understanding the risks of the procedure involved and risks attached to rejecting the available procedure" [13]. Nine participants in the research had lesions that progressed to invasive cancer, and 62 women developed carcinoma in situ of the cervix [25]; this means they needed to be enrolled for treatment, since the fundamental principles that guide decisions in biomedical research highlight respect for persons, beneficence, and justice. Moreover, Peppercorn et al. [26] argue that when the guidelines are respected, an informed adult with cancer can both understand and voluntarily consent to participation in a clinical trial involving mandatory research biopsy.

Cancer surveillance may also require the viewing of archived health information of civilians attending government-controlled health facilities or information on the deceased kept at the government-controlled mortuaries. In these cases, consent from patients or relatives (family) may not be regarded as important as researchers often regard this kind of research as posing less or no harm to those involved. They then justify their actions by pointing to low response rate evidence often associated with giving too much detail [26, 27] and by suggesting that this research will not result in harm to the individuals in question. Corti et al. [28] have emphasized the importance of anonymization and of methods of gate-keeping for access to archived data in an effort to protect the rights of participants who authorized that their data be stored. They further argue that the people concerned be re-contacted to procure valid consent.

Moreover, because community surveys include a large number of community participants (involving large budgets that developing countries cannot afford), a larger number of fieldworkers are needed and often less-specialized individuals are employed (since they will be regarded as cheap labour—to cut costs) to collect data and sometimes perform specialized screening procedures. Although these individuals tend to be "extensively" trained to conduct the procedures, they may not be registered to any health profession body, and as such cannot be regulated. This is a major ethical breach, since these individuals are not being trained to conduct "best practice research." Clear example of this kind of ethical breach was found in a study conducted in Brazil by Marodin et al. [29], which suggested that fieldworkers were returning results that were not clinically validated, as they had no medical-practice background.

Privacy is the right to be free from unwanted intrusion into one's personal life, while confidentiality is the right to be free from unwanted disclosure of personal information, as this can cause stigma, stress, and insecurity, and sometimes, physical harm. Thus, in research, personal information needs to be kept as confidential as possible, a principle that is very often broken, as discussed by Corti et al. [28]. They pose deep concerns regarding the rights of participants that are often breached with issues of confidentiality and informed consent violated during archiving qualitative material. In practice, confidentiality assurance implies no collection of personal information unless necessary, avoiding non-intended disclosures, keeping all collected data anonymous wherever possible, and no disclosure of identifying information without the participant's consent.

Keeping data anonymous sometimes poses a serious challenge. One would use, for example, anonymous questionnaires whenever possible, encrypted codes as identifiers in database and in analysis datasets, and keep a separate master-list with identifying information and decryption codes, only accessible to the investigator. Nonetheless, Naam and Sanbar [30] observe that with advanced technology including electronic communication and social media, maintaining patient's confidentiality could prove extremely difficult. The requirement for database and source documents to only be accessible via strict access codes may not always be realizable [26].

Beneficence and Non-Maleficence

Most medical breakthroughs (chemotherapy, in particular) have come from clinical research. However, such research sometimes has tragic outcomes because it may expose participants to harm/maltreatment. Although it is very rare that participants become harmed or even die while taking part in clinical trials, it has to be noted that all research carries some risk. The risk of unwanted disclosure and potential harm is always there. Furthermore, not all risks can be foreseen and the probability or magnitude of harm cannot always be assessed. Thus, a researcher should exhibit an ethical attitude and sensitivity to the special needs of individual participants in addition to providing high standards of healthcare [31].

Furthermore, the protection of participants requires approval of study by an ethics committee and ethics oversight during study implementation. The role of research ethics committees is to review research on human subjects. The committee is supposed to assume the role of protecting dependent and vulnerable research subjects within the research process [32].

In fact, Lallemant and Le Coeur [33] in their review of complex scientific and ethical issues raised by clinical trials emphasized that researchers need to ensure that populations in less economically developed situations that accept the risk of the research receive the full benefit of that research and that the vaccine, if proven successful, be made accessible and affordable to them.

Participant protection expects from the researcher careful monitoring and treatment of any foreseen and unforeseen adverse events, fast reporting of adverse events to the ethics committee, stopping the study if safety concerns dictate, providing compensation for injuries to the participant [14, 18].

Research may contribute towards advanced physiological and epidemiological understanding of disease, or toward new or improved tools for prevention, screening or diagnosis, and treatment. Yet, the researcher sometimes faces the challenge of offering the patient the most beneficial treatment available while fulfilling the obligation to use rigorous experimental methods, including randomized controlled trials to discover what is best for patients generally, including the investigation of experimental modalities. To deal with this equipoise problem, a researcher should be able to strike a balance between the ethical obligations to patients and the need for scientific and public health advances [29].

Conflict of interest is another issue related to justice of study subjects. A conflict of interest has the potential to undermine the integrity of scientific research as well as to threaten public trust in scientific findings [28]. Substantial rewards may come to researchers at the end of a research project, such as renewed funding, academic promotion, salary increases, increased respect from colleagues, and in some cases, fame and fortune. In light of this, the welfare of the individual subjects of research may be sacrificed or compromised due to these competing interests. Solutions to conflict of interest include disclosure of conflicts of interest and self-removal from situations where conflict exists [28].

For instance, Kass et al. [15] have highlighted issues regarding conflict of interest in developing countries (Africa, in particular) where funding obtained from non-reputable sources compromised the integrity of cancer researchers, such that the trust in their scientific findings was questioned. Other potential conflicts were also raised regarding the ability of cancer research reviewers to avoid conflicts. For instance, reviewers experienced unease voicing objections when fellow members' protocols were reviewed, fearing being labelled unfriendly. Moreover, community members who were also RERC panel members were reluctant to reject protocols believed to bring employment. Finally, protocols that were viewed as bringing income to the institution did not undergo intensive review and were cleared quickly by RERCs.

Justice

Justice in research is another basic ethical principle prescribing fair distribution of the burdens and benefits of research involving human subjects among all layers of the society.

Selection of participants should be fair, with persons being selected only because of the specific subject area being studied, and not because of their easy availability or their reduced autonomy [30].

Vulnerable persons are all those who have diminished ability to protect their own interests, those with reduced capacity to give informed consent, incapacity to understand or communicate, or who are not in a position to make a voluntary decision. These vulnerable persons include prisoners, children, pregnant women, mentally disabled, terminally ill patients [8, 14, 18].

The CIOMS Guidelines recommend standards for the application of the Helsinki guidelines in developing countries, as research integrity is a problem in the developing world such as in Africa [31]. This includes stipulations that research products be made reasonably available to the inhabitants of any host developing country. The Declaration of Helsinki, article 25 states: "When a subject deemed legally incompetent, such as a minor child, is able to give assent to decisions about participation in research, the investigator must obtain that assent in addition to the consent of the legally authorized representative" [14]. Moreover, Markman [34] has since emphasized that, under no circumstances should a study ever be permitted to satisfy regulatory requirements for licensing approval in the "developed" world if there is reliable evidence that *any* of the human subjects entered into that trial were not treated with adequate safeguards, or that ethically mandated informed consent procedures designed to respect the autonomy and dignity of all people were not employed. This is in response to the fact that minors (boys and girls) and vulnerable individuals from low-resourced communities are often included in cancer procedures endorsed by western pharmaceutical companies, without even being given a chance to benefit from those procedures.

Researchers have the obligation to be sensitive to the special nature of these individuals. Special justification will be required to invite such persons to participate in research. The CIOMS Guidelines require that additional safeguards be employed to protect their rights and welfare. This may involve limits to the amount of risk allowed, consent provided by proxy or surrogate decision making that utilizes the best interests standard, consent monitors as well as the on-going monitoring of research, and non-coercion [10, 11, 23]. The next section will discuss the issues of plagiarism, forgery, and the falsification of data.

Plagiarism, Forgery, and the Falsification of Data (Results in Developing Countries)

Scientific misconduct is often motivated by the issue of "publish or perish" that often leads to career pressure—where desperate (or fame-hungry) scientists tend to fabricate (make up) results, falsify (manipulate) results, or conduct plagiarism (use other people's ideas without giving appropriate credit). The issues of misconduct are not unique to developing countries [35]; however, developing countries often fall into the trap due to various reasons ranging from: (1) difficulty in writing for English language journals, which can tempt researchers to plagiarize text; (2) pressures exerted by their non-reputable funders; and, (3) institutions with hunger for output, such that scientists in those institutions experience pressures to maintain their career in research. In a study conducted by Ana et al. [36] to evaluate the extent of dishonest behavior in biomedicine in developing countries, it was observed that, with the exception of China, which has created an office of scientific research integrity, scientific misconduct is rife in the other developing countries and is most common in the poor nations as they are inadequately prepared to take action against this misconduct. For example, Ana et al. [35] cite a case where between 1991 and 1999, an oncologist working at the University of Witwatersrand in Johannesburg, South Africa, treated thousands of women suffering from breast cancer with bone transplantations. Werner Bezwoda reported amazing results with 90 % of his patients achieving complete remission. But an independent study with contradictory results had concerns, since the trial records had been manipulated. To combat scientific misconduct, Ana et al. [36] highlight the need for both institutional and national systems in developing countries to regulate and control biomedical research. They also highlight the fact that research partners and research funding agencies should take a greater interest in research misconduct, or in supporting the development and strengthening of national platforms, policies, and procedures to address it.

Okonta and Rossouw [37] also conducted a study to investigate attitudes and perceptions towards misconduct in a group of researchers in Nigeria. Their findings suggested that half of their respondents were aware of a colleague who had committed misconduct; over 88 % of the researchers were concerned about the perceived amount of misconduct prevalent in their institution; while the majority believed that the chance of getting caught for scientific misconduct in their work environment was low.

Summary

This chapter outlines ethical issues in developing countries, with a particular focus on the challenges experienced by the RERCs in these countries. These challenges emanate from budget constraints experienced by governments making it difficult for them to support cancer research, resulting in shortcomings in full review and regulation of cancer research. As such, several issues of misconduct by cancer researchers arise. These range from: (1) the rights of participants being violated, such that the issues of confidentiality, fair participant selection, and informed consent are overlooked; with (2) the professional integrity of researchers compromised, when researchers receive research funding from non-reputable sources; moreover, (3) scientific misconduct also motivated by the issue of "publish or perish" that often leads to career pressure with researchers tending to fabricate and falsify cancer research results or conduct plagiarism. These ethics issues are not unique to developing countries; however, governments in developing countries need to put cancer research at the forefront of the political agenda so as to advance the quality of cancer research, also enforcing researcher compliance with international laws and other requirements for research that involves human subjects. Moreover, the complexities in cancer research in developing countries encourage the development of the country-specific practical guide to cancer research.

References

1. GLOBOCAN 2012. Estimated cancer incidence, mortality and prevalence worldwide in 2012. 2012. http://globocan.iarc.fr/Pages/summary_table_pop_sel.aspx. Accessed 2 May 2015.
2. Vin-Raviv N, Akinyemiju TF, Galea S, Bovbjerg DH. Depression and anxiety disorders among hospitalized women with breast cancer. PLoS One. 2015;10(6), e0129169.
3. Duska LR, Dizon DS. Improving quality of life in female cancer survivors: current status and future questions. Future Oncol. 2014;10(6):1015–26.
4. Hodhodinezhad N, Zahedi R, Ashrafi-rizzi H, Shams A. A scientometric study of general internal medicine domain among Muslim countries of middle East (1991–2011). Acta Inform Med. 2013;21(1):55–9.
5. Shao H, Yu Q, Bo X, Duan Z. Analysis of oncology research from 2001 to 2010: a scientometric perspective. Oncol Rep. 2013;29(4):1441–52. Epub 2013 Jan 17.
6. Kirigia JM, Wambebe C. Status of national health research systems in ten countries of the WHO African Region. BMC Health Serv Res. 2006;6:135.
7. CDC. The public health system and the 10 essential public health services. 2015. http://www. cdc.gov/nphpsp/essentialServices.html. Accessed 5 May 2015.
8. International Network for Cancer Treatment and Research. Cancer in developing countries. 2015. http://www.inctr.org/about-inctr/cancer-in-developing-countries. Accessed on 5 May 2015.

9. Adebamowo CA, Akarolo-Anthony S. Cancer in Africa: opportunities for collaborative research and training. Afr J Med Sci. 2009;38 Suppl 2:5–13.
10. World Health Organization. International agency for research on cancer. 2015. http://www.iarc.fr/index.php. Accessed on 2 Mar 2015.
11. Murray SA, Grant E, Grant A, Kendall M. Dying from cancer in developed and developing countries: lessons from two qualitative interview studies of patients and their carers. BMJ. 2003;326:368.
12. Steyn NP, Mchiza ZJ. Obesity and the nutrition transition in Sub-Saharan Africa. Ann NY Acad Sci. 2014;1311:88–101.
13. Levine RJ (Ed.). The Belmont report: ethical principles and guidelines for the protection of human subjects. Appendix 11. The National Commission for the Protection of Human Subjects of Biomedical and Behavioral Research. DHEW Publication No. (OS) 78–0014. http://videocast.nih.gov/pdf/ohrp_appendix_belmont_report_vol_2.pdf. Accessed on 2 Mar 2015.
14. Bartlett EE. International analysis of institutional review boards registered with the U.S. office for Human Research Protection. J Empir Res Hum Res Ethics. 2008;3(4):49–56.
15. Kass NE, Hyder AA, Ajuwon A, et al. The structure and function of research ethics committees in Africa: a case study. PLoS Med. 2007;4(1):0026–31 (open access). http://www.plosmedicine.org/article/fetchObject.action?uri=info:doi/10.1371/journal.pmed.0040003&representation=PDF. Accessed 12 Feb 2015.
16. Rivera R, Ezcurra E. Composition and operation of selected research ethics review committees in Latin America. IRB. 2001;23:9–12.
17. US Department of Health and Human Services (DHHS); Public Health Service; National Institutes of Health. OPRR Reports, code of federal regulations 45CFR46 and certain other related laws and regulations in protection of human subjects. Bethesda, MD: National Institutes of Health. 1983.
18. The Norwegian National Committees for Research Ethics. General guidelines for research ethics. 2015. https://www.etikkom.no/en/research-ethical-guidelines/general-guidelines-for-research-ethics/. Accessed 2 Mar 2015.
19. Verástegui EL. Consenting of the vulnerable: the informed consent procedure in advanced cancer patients in Mexico. BMC Med Ethics. 2006;7, E13.
20. Ali R, Finlayson A; Indox Cancer Research Network. Building capacity for clinical research in developing countries: the INDOX Cancer Research Network experience. Glob Health Action. 2012;5. doi: 10.3402/gha.v5i0.17288. Epub 2012 May 2.
21. University of Minnesota Center for Bioethics. A guide to research ethics. 2003. http://www.ahc.umn.edu/img/assets/26104/Research_Ethics.pdf. Accessed 2 Mar 2015.
22. Council for International Organizations of Medical Sciences; WHO. International ethical guidelines for biomedical research involving human subjects. 2002. http://www.cioms.ch/publications/layout_guide2002.pdf. Accessed 3 Mar 2015.
23. Courser MW. The impact of active consent procedures on nonresponse and nonresponse error in youth survey data: evidence from a new experiment. Eval Rev. 2009;33(4):370–95. doi:10.1177/0193841X09337228.
24. Sadetzki S, Langer CE, Bruchim R, et al. The MOBI-kids study protocol: challenges in assessing childhood and adolescent exposure to electromagnetic fields from wireless telecommunication technologies and possible association with brain tumor risk. Front Public Health. 2014;2:124. doi:10.3389/fpubh.2014.00124. eCollection 2014.
25. Mudur G. Indian study of women with cervical lesions called unethical. BMJ. 1997;314(7087):1065.
26. Peppercorn J, Shapira I, Collyar D, et al. Ethics of mandatory research biopsy for correlative end points within clinical trials in oncology. J Clin Oncol. 2010;28(15):2635–40. doi:10.1200/JCO.2009.27.2443. Epub 2010 Apr 20.
27. Bolcic-Jankovic D, Clarridge BR, Fowler Jr FJ. Consent forms affect the response rate? Alexandria: AAPOR—ASA Section on Survey Research Methods; 2005. p. 3810–4.

28. Corti L, Day A, Backhouse G. Confidentiality and informed consent: issues for consideration in the preservation of and provision of access to qualitative data archives [46 paragraphs]. Forum qualitative sozialforschung/forum: qualitative social research, 1(3), Art. 7. 2000. http://nbn-resolving.de/urn:nbn:de:0114-fqs000372. Accessed 2 Mar 2015.
29. Marodin G, França P, Rocha JC, Campos AH. Biobanking for health research in Brazil: present challenges and future directions. Rev Panam Salud Publica. 2012;31(6):523–8.
30. Naam NH, Sanbar S. Advanced technology and confidentiality in hand surgery. J Hand Surg Am. 2015;40(1):182–7. doi:10.1016/j.jhsa.2014.03.011.
31. Kleiderman E, Avard D, Black L, Diaz Z, Rousseau C, Knoppers BM. Recruiting terminally Ill patients into non-therapeutic oncology studies: views of health professionals. BMC Med Ethics. 2012;13:33.
32. Truman C. Ethics and the ruling relations of research production. Paper 1. Social Sciences. 2003. http://digitalcommons.bolton.ac.uk/socsci_journalspr/1. Accessed 2 Mar 2015.
33. Lallemant M, Le Coeur S. Clinical experimentation with HIV vaccines: scientific and ethical dilemmas. Hist Philos Life Sci. 1995;17(1):151–69.
34. Markman M. Assuring the ethical conduct of clinical cancer trials in the developing world. Cancer. 2006;106(1):1–3.
35. Resnik DB. Research ethics timeline (1932–Present). National Institute of Environmental Health. Your environment, your health. 2015. http://www.niehs.nih.gov/research/resources/bioethics/timeline/. Accessed 2 Mar 2015.
36. Ana J, Koehlmoos T, Smith R, Yan LL. Research misconduct in low- and middle-income countries. PLoS Med. 2013;10(3):1–6.e1001315.
37. Okonta PI, Rossouw T. Misconduct in research: a descriptive survey of attitudes, perceptions and associated factors in a developing country. BMC Med Ethics. 2014;15:25.
38. Marzouk D, Abd El Aal W, Saleh A, Sleem H, Khyatti M, Mazini L, Hemminki K, Anwar WA. Overview on health research ethics in Egypt and North Africa. Eur J Public Health. 2014;24 Suppl 1:87–91. doi:10.1093/eurpub/cku110.
39. Mano MS, Rosa DD, Dal LL. Multinational clinical trials in oncology and post-trial benefits for host countries: where do we stand? Eur J Cancer. 2006;42(16):2675–7. Epub 2006 Sep 7.
40. Markman M. An ethical argument in support of interactions between developing world countries and pharmaceutical/biotechnology companies involved in oncology drug development. Cancer. 2008;112(9):1871–3. doi:10.1002/cncr.23385.
41. Prasai S. Human papilloma virus vaccination: should it be mandatory? J Nepal Med Assoc. 2008;47(171):167–71.
42. Simon C, Mosavel M, van Stade D. Ethical challenges in the design and conduct of locally relevant international health research. Soc Sci Med. 2007;64(9):1960–9. doi:10.1016/j.socscimed.2007.01.009.
43. Natunen K, Lehtinen J, Namujju P, Sellors J, Lehtinen M. Aspects of prophylactic vaccination against cervical cancer and other human papillomavirus-related cancers in developing countries. Infect Dis Obstet Gynecol. 2011;2011:675858. doi:10.1155/2011/675858. Epub 2011 Jul 19.
44. Tomljenovic L, Shaw CA. Human papillomavirus (HPV) vaccine policy and evidence-based medicine: are they at odds? Ann Med. 2013;45(2):182–93. doi:10.3109/07853890.2011.645353. Epub 2011 Dec 22.

Chapter 7
Data Management and Statistics

Jingmei Jiang, Philip C. Nasca, Wei Han, Fang Xue, and Biao Zhang

Abstract Data management refers to a set of procedures including the collection, integration, and validation of research data. As an essential part of research, data management is necessary in order to obtain accurate and reliable data, to ensure research integrity and replication, to conduct the research in an efficient manner, to ensure the security of data, and finally to comply with regulatory requirements/guidelines.

Thus, data management is a multidisciplinary activity and involves staff with different professional backgrounds (e.g., principal investigator (PI), data administrator, data monitor, and statistician).

The essential elements of data management are represented by design of collection form, data base designs, data entry, data storage and security, data coding, and data validation.

Keywords Data management • Statistics • Test validity • Sensitivity • Specificity • Quality control • Positive and negative predictive value • Age-standardized rate • Linear regression

Abbreviations

ASR	Age-standardized rate
AUC	Area under the ROC curve
CI	Confidence interval
CIN2+	Moderate or severe cervical intraepithelial neoplasia or cancer
CMH	Cochrane–Mantel–Hansel
CRF	Case report form

J. Jiang, Ph.D. (✉) • W. Han, Ph.D. • F. Xue, Ph.D. • B. Zhang, Ph.D.
Department of Epidemiology and Statistics, Institute of Basic Medical Sciences,
Chinese Academy of Medical Sciences and School of Basic Medicine,
Peking Union Medical College, 5 Dong Dan San Tiao, Beijing 100005, China
e-mail: jingmeijiang@ibms.pumc.edu.cn

P.C. Nasca, Ph.D.
School of Public Health, State University of New York, USA

© Springer International Publishing Switzerland 2016
D.C. Stefan (ed.), *Cancer Research and Clinical Trials in Developing Countries*, DOI 10.1007/978-3-319-18443-2_7

CUMI	Cumulative incidence
DF	Degree of freedom
DMP	Data management plan
FNR	False negative rate
FPR	False positive rate
GCP	Good clinical practice
HC2	The digene high-risk HPV HC2 DNA
HR	Hazard ratio
ICD-10-CM	International Classification of Diseases, Tenth Revision, Clinical Modification
ICH	International Conference on Harmonization of Technical Requirements for Registration of Pharmaceuticals for Human Use
KM	Kaplan–Meier
LBC	Liquid-based cytology
LR	Likelihood ratio
LR+	The likelihood ratio for a positive test
LR−	The likelihood ratio for a negative test
MedDRA	Medical Dictionary for Regulatory Activities
NPV	Negative predictive value
OR	Odds ratio
PI	Principal investigator
PPV	Positive predictive value
ROC	Receiver operating characteristic
RR	Rate ratio
Se	Sensitivity
SE	Standard error
Sp	Specificity
SRR	Standardized rate ratio
TASR	Truncated age-standardized rate
TNR	True negative rate
TPR	True positive rate
WHO-DDE	World Health Organization-Drug Dictionary Enhanced

Introduction

Clinical cancer research encompasses large, complex, and systematic studies, which are mainly concerned with the prevention, diagnosis, and treatment of cancer. Sound data management and appropriate statistical analysis, as indispensable parts of clinical cancer research, are critical to ensure the integrity of the research, as well as supporting the hypotheses, and giving credibility to research conclusions.

In this chapter, we introduce fundamental data management principles and conventional statistical approaches applicable to analysis conducted in the clinical cancer research field. To illustrate the statistical method for easier comprehension, several cancer research studies conducted in China are incorporated as examples. We do not intend to replace statistics reference books. Our objective is solely to assist readers to conduct clinical cancer research when dealing with data requiring statistical and quantitative analysis, by providing an overview of data management and statistical methods.

Data Management in Clinical Cancer Research

Clinical cancer research can be classified into observational research (e.g., case–control study, cohort study) and experimental research (e.g., clinical trial), with regard to interventions (treatments) imposed on the patient during the research process. No matter what the type of research, all studies face common problems: how to obtain high-quality data and how to perform this process efficiently. Data management refers to a set of procedures including the collection, integration, and validation of research data. As an essential part of research, data management is necessary: (1) to obtain accurate and reliable data; (2) to ensure research integrity and replication; (3) to conduct the research in an efficient manner; (4) to ensure the security of data; and, (5) to comply with regulatory requirements/guidelines. Thus, data management is a multidisciplinary activity and involves staff with different professional backgrounds (e.g., principal investigator (PI), data administrator, data monitor, and statistician).

In this section, we will introduce some fundamental data-management issues in clinical cancer research, as well as Good Clinical Practice (GCP) guidelines that should be complied with when conducting clinical trials. In addition, data management for cancer registration is also introduced because of its importance in cancer prevention and control.

Essential Elements of Data Management

The essential elements in the workflow of data management are presented in Fig. 7.1, and these are shared by most types of clinical research. However, variations may exist either in the structure of the workflow or in the implementation of a

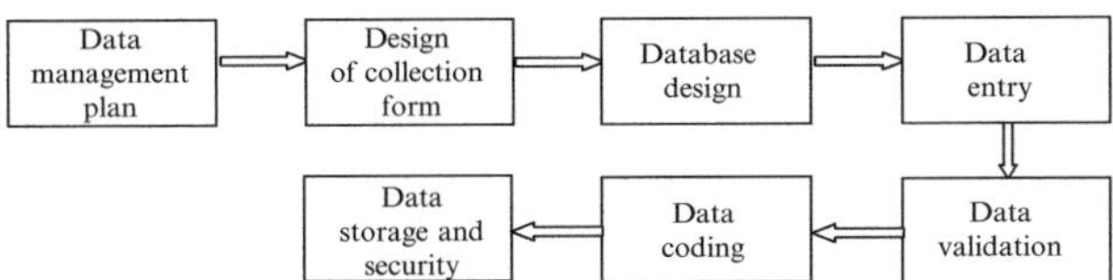

Fig. 7.1 Flow chart of data management

specific step in the workflow for different types of cancer research. For instance, in clinical trials, data management may be more complicated and some special issues (e.g., the maintenance of essential trial documents for audit and serious adverse event reporting) should be dealt with to meet the requirements of the regulatory authority.

Data Management Plan

The objective of creating a data management plan (DMP) is to help the researcher to manage the data in a systematic and efficient manner and to ensure that data management meets the requirements of the project funder or relevant authority overseeing the research. Thus, a DMP should list all the necessary elements and personnel required for data management in a specific study, such as research information, data types and structure, specific data-management practice, and confidentiality issues.

Design of Data Collection Form

The data collection form is of major importance in a research study because, as an illustration of the study protocol, it determines what data should be collected in the study process.

The most commonly used data-collection tool in clinical research is the Case Report Form (CRF) and it can be constructed through three steps: item identification, draft composition, and CRF validation, which are presented in Fig. 7.2.

1. Item identification: Necessary items can be identified by reviewing the protocol to achieve the study objectives and meet regulatory requirements.
2. Draft composition: Items identified should be phrased in an appropriate way, which is called item design. The objective is to make the questions clear and concise, so that they can be answered unambiguously and efficiently. Then, the layout of items should be organized, and a structural order reflecting the time points that data are collected is suggested for this process.
3. CRF validation: The CRF should be validated before being put into use to ensure its quality, which is usually done by pretesting it in a pilot study. In addition, it is best to have the CRF reviewed by experienced researchers, data managers, and statisticians.

Fig. 7.2 CRF design process

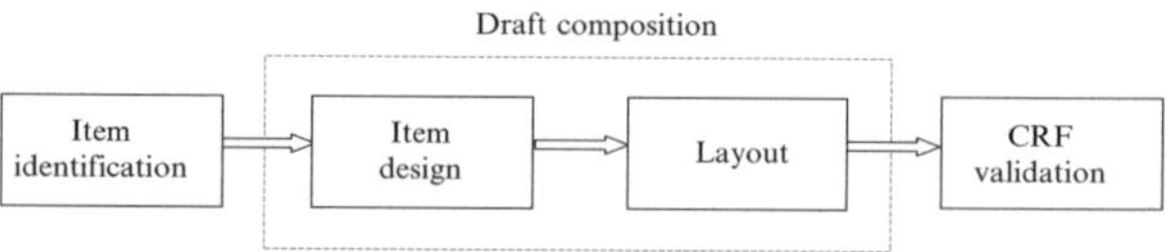

Database Design

A database is a structured set of data that allows for complicated data cleaning, reviewing, and reporting. The ultimate goal of database design is to store data accurately, that is, the contents of the database should accurately reflect the observations of the research. To meet these requirements, the database should be constructed in accordance with the study protocol or CRF and allow convenient data entry. The database should also support internal checks, so that problems can be detected in a timely manner.

Data Entry

The basic rule for transcribing data from data-collection forms to database is to reduce errors in data entry to a minimum. In most cases, data should be entered twice to ensure data quality and minimize the error rate. It has been shown that the error rate can be as low as 0.001 % if the double entry method is employed. Data entry can be performed either by professional data entry staff or data coordinators or other staff who are familiar with the research.

Data entry can be done at each participant site where data were collected or in a data coordinating center after all the data have been received. For multicenter clinical research, Electronic Data Capture (EDC) systems are usually implemented because they enable the immediate entry at the participant site and facilitate the data transfer process. EDC is the trend for clinical data collection for multicenters, especially for developing countries, although its usage is still at low level.

Data Validation

Errors are inevitable in the data transfer process (for example, the filling of CRF, data entry, and data export). Data validation refers to the steps in finding the errors in collected data in accordance with the protocol specifications. For instance, completeness checks, range checks for outliners, logical inconsistences, and protocol violations.

Data-validation procedures mainly include: source data verification process (checking consistence between data in CRF with source data at the research site by data monitor) and data cleaning (checking the accuracy and validity by probing errors for data submitted to the data-management team). An automatic check by an editing computer program is the most common and reliable method for data validation, and most errors can be detected automatically.

Data Coding

Data collected in the form of text is often encountered in clinical cancer research, for example, adverse events, medical history, diagnoses, and medicine use information. To make data in text forms appropriate for analysis, some rules should be created in advance or existing medical dictionaries should be implemented to replace text with code. The most commonly used medical dictionaries include: Medical Dictionary for Regulatory Activities (MedDRA), which is used for the coding of adverse events and other illnesses; the International Classification of Diseases, Tenth Revision, Clinical Modification (ICD-10-CM), which is used for coding diseases such as relevant history, concomitant diseases, and cause of death; and the World Health Organization-Drug Dictionary Enhanced (WHO-DDE), which is used for coding drug use.

Data Storage and Security

Storage of research data in an appropriate manner can facilitate its management and assessment. There are several options for storing data, such as networked drives, personal computers, and external storage devices (e.g., hard drives and USB flash drives). It is highly recommended that research data be stored on regularly backed-up networked drives in the research center. This ensures that research data are stored in a relatively secure place and backed up regularly. The use of personal computers and external storage devices carries the risk of the devices and data being lost or stolen.

Data security refers to the protection of research data during the research process, and the best way is to limit internal and external access to the data. PIs should decide which project members are authorized to access and manage the stored data. Documents and CRFs should be kept in a safe, secure location away from public access. For digital research data, additional attention should be paid to safeguarding the data, e.g., implementing anti-virus protection and using a firewall, recording the original creation date and time for files in the system, using encryption, electronic signatures, or watermarking to keep track of authorship and changes to data files, and regularly backing up electronic data files.

Quality Control for Data Management

Errors can arise at each stage in the research process, from data collection to transcription into the database. Unreliable information is worse than no information because unreliable information could bias the research conclusions. The value of the research is greatly influenced by quality control, which refers to a set of operational activities conducted at each stage of the research process to ensure the quality of data and to verify that research is carried out in accordance with the study protocol and the standard operating procedures.

Quality control can be a component of routine data management work, such as CRF validation, staff training, and keeping records of daily research activities in the form of a data-management document. It can also be an activity that is specially designed to ensure the quality of data management, e.g., checks for completeness and consistency between data in the CRF and source data, and cleaning of data entered into the database. In most cases, a data monitor is responsible for performing the quality control checks by: (1) reviewing data management documentation to assess adherence to written procedures, policies, and regulations; and, (2) detecting inconsistencies and errors through review of data collection forms.

Good Clinical Practice in Clinical Trials

Guidelines for high-quality research are required for clinical trials, which focus on testing the safety and efficacy of specific drugs or devices that require approval by the relevant agency for commercial use. GCP, provided by the International Conference on Harmonization of Technical Requirements for Registration of Pharmaceuticals for Human Use (ICH), is an international quality standard for designing, conducting, recording, and reporting trials that involve the participation of human subjects. Compliance with this standard can ensure that the rights, safety, and well-being of trial subjects are protected.

The baseline standards of ICH-GCP have acquired agreement worldwide. However, the specific implementation varies for different nations. For example, in the United States, the Food and Drug Administration monitors the conduct of clinical trials, and regulations governing their conduct in the United States are in the Code of Federal Regulations. Some developing countries have put forward their own GCP guidelines in consideration of the actual situation in their countries. When the ICH-GCP is implemented in developing countries, some considerations should be made to tailor them adequately because of the context-specific difficulties such as the socioeconomic vulnerability of the study population, logistical constraints, and weaknesses in the regulatory framework and ethics approval system.

Data Management in Cancer Registration

Cancer registration refers to the collection of clinical and pathological characteristics of a particular cancer continuously and systematically in a defined population. It is helpful for monitoring the status and changes in cancer occurrence at the population level, clinical decision making, and defining priorities in cancer prevention and care.

There are two kinds of cancer registration: population-based cancer registration and hospital-based cancer registration, which have different objectives and data sources. In this section, we mainly discuss population-based cancer registration because of its value in obtaining the incidence of cancer in the general population.

Cancer registration can collect cancer data from various sources, such as private clinics, general practitioners, laboratories, hospices, health insurance systems, screening programs, and central registers, and the data-collection process can be done in an active or passive way, which differs in whether the cancer registration personnel actually visit the sources of data and abstract the required information. Three kinds of information are crucial for collecting information from these sources: personal identification information (e.g., name, sex, birth date); demographic information (e.g., address of usual residence, nationality, ethnic group); and tumor information (e.g., date of diagnosis, behavior, most valid method of diagnosis, source of information, clinical stage). ICD-Oncology is recommended when classifying neoplasm information because it can provide optimal facilities for coding and reporting cancers and uses the behavior, topography, and histological details of the cancer in the coding process.

Quality control for cancer registration plays an important role just as it does in clinical cancer research, and they share some common basic requirements (e.g., reliability and accuracy). However, some special issues should be addressed for cancer registration data, which are: (1) completeness: the registration actually contains cases it is supposed to contain and does not contain other "cases"; and, (2) timeliness: data collection must be conducted according to the schedule. Details of quality control strategies for cancer registration can be found in the series of publications by the North American Association of Central Cancer Registries [1].

The role of cancer registration in developing countries should not be overlooked. However, it may not be realistic to establish cancer registries that are as complex as those in developed countries because of the lack of the necessary infrastructure. Other factors also threaten the establishment of cancer registration, such as unavailability of nominative death records, lack of trained personnel, inaccurate population data, cultural taboos, political or economic instability, and massive population movements. Thus, data management in cancer registration should be adapted to conditions with limited resources in developing countries. For instance, information collection work should focus on data items that are essential for registration, and emphasis should be placed on ensuring the completeness and quality of the data. In addition, active data-collection methods should play a more important role in the data-collection process because the medical infrastructure might be underdeveloped.

Statistical Methods for Cancer Screening and Diagnostic Tests

In the process of cancer prevention and control, secondary prevention, i.e., early discovery, early diagnosis, and early treatment of cancers, plays a very important role, because it directly influences the prognosis, survival rate, and mortality of patients. Screening and diagnostic tests, as two important clinical tools for detecting or confirming disease, may greatly enhance the level of cancer prevention and control [2, 3]. Therefore, it is necessary for the clinician and related researchers to be familiar with basic concepts, evaluation indicators, and methods in both screening and diagnostic tests.

Screening and Diagnostic Tests

The screening test (1957) was defined by the United States Commission on Chronic Illness as: "the presumptive identification of unrecognized disease or defect by the application of tests, examinations or other procedures that can be applied rapidly" [4]. It mainly aims to classify asymptomatic people as likely or unlikely to have disease early, for early diagnosis, early treatment, and a better prognosis.

In clinical cancer research, an effective cancer-screening program should follow four important principles: (1) the cancer to be screened should be an important health problem, and the cause of substantial mortality and/or morbidity; (2) the cancer should have a detectable preclinical phase; (3) therapy initiated as a result of cancer being detected by screening should be effective; and, (4) the cancer-screening method should be acceptable and safe. In the past several decades, some cancer-screening programs, such as cervix, breast, colorectal, lung, and prostate, had been successfully carried out in many developed countries and some developing countries, which improved the prognostic greatly and lowered the incidence and mortality [5–7].

A diagnostic test is the process of identifying patients with a disease or condition by assessing the signs, symptoms, and results of objective laboratory tests. The presence or absence of disease can be ultimately ascertained by a gold standard method, which often refers to a biopsy, surgical exploration, or autopsy, etc.

The relationship between screening and diagnosis tests is presented in Fig. 7.3. Although screening and diagnostic tests have different target populations and test purposes, they share some common evaluation indicators and analytic methods.

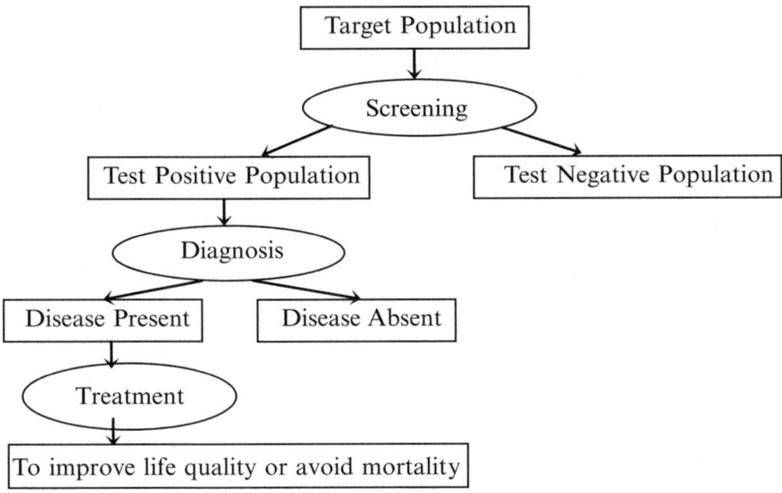

Fig. 7.3 Flow chart of the screening and diagnosis of diseases

Evaluation of Test Validity

One of the crucial aspects for assessing screening and diagnostic tests is its validity, which refers to the ability of a test to correctly detect a condition when it is actually present and to correctly rule out a condition when it is truly absent. Two important measures of test validity are sensitivity and specificity, which describe how well the test performs compared to a gold standard test.

Sensitivity and Specificity

The characteristics of sensitivity and specificity can be expressed in a 2×2 contingency table (Table 7.1).

1. Sensitivity (Se) is the probability of testing positive given the presence of disease, it is estimated using following formula:

$$\mathrm{Se} = \frac{\text{Number who test positive with a disease}\left(a\right)}{\text{Number with a disease}\left(a+c\right)} \times 100\ \% \tag{7.1}$$

   It can also be called the true positive rate (TPR) in a diagnostic test.

2. Specificity (Sp) is the probability of testing negative given the absence of disease, it is estimated using following formula:

$$\mathrm{Sp} = \frac{\text{Number who test negative without a disease}\left(d\right)}{\text{Number without a disease}\left(b+d\right)} \times 100\ \% \tag{7.2}$$

   It can also be called the true negative rate (TNR) in a diagnostic test.
   Sensitivity and specificity, as measures of intrinsic diagnostic validity, are not affected by the prevalence of the disease.
   There are also two other indicators for measuring validity.

3. False-positive rate (FPR) is the probability of testing positive given the absence of disease, it is estimated using following formula:

$$\mathrm{FPR} = \frac{\text{Number who test positive without a disease}\left(b\right)}{\text{Number without a disease}\left(b+d\right)} \times 100\ \% \tag{7.3}$$

   It corresponds to TPR.

Table 7.1 Basic 2×2 count table

Test result	True condition status	
	Present	Absent
Positive	a	b
Negative	c	d

$a, b, c,$ and d represent the frequency in each cell

Table 7.2 Relationship between TPR, TNR, FNR, and FPR

Test result	True condition status	
	Present	Absent
Positive	TPR $a/(a+c)$	FPR $b/(b+d)$
Negative	FNR $c/(a+c)$	TNR $d/(b+d)$

4. False-negative rate (FNR) is the probability of testing negative given the presence of disease, it is estimated using following formula:

$$\text{FNR} = \frac{\text{Number who test negative with a disease}(c)}{\text{Number with a disease}(a+c)} \times 100\ \%$$ (7.4)

It corresponds to TNR.

Thus, Table 7.1 can also be expressed as Table 7.2.

Obviously, TPR + FNR = 1 and TNR + FPR = 1, which indicates that the best way to reduce FNR and FPR simultaneously is to maximize the TPR and TNR.

In clinical practice, a highly sensitive test is usually used when there is an important penalty for missing a disease. For instance, a false negative will lead to delays in diagnosis and treatment. On the other hand, a highly specific test is usually needed when a false positive can harm patients physically, emotionally, or financially by suffering a great risk of confirmatory test. Therefore, a high-quality cancer screening and diagnostic test should balance the need for sensitivity and specificity in the specific circumstance.

Because sensitivity and specificity are proportional indicators, standard errors (SEs) and confidence intervals (CIs) can be estimated. When the sample size is large, SE and CI of both Se and Sp can be calculated in accordance with the normal approximation theorem, using SE and CI of proportions. Only formulae for Se are given here. Calculation formulae for other indicators are similar.

SE of Se can be calculated as follow:

$$\text{SE}(\text{Se}) = \sqrt{\frac{\text{Se}(1-\text{Se})}{a+c}} = \sqrt{\frac{ac}{(a+c)^3}}$$ (7.5)

$100(1-\alpha)\%$ CI for Se can be obtained:

$$\left(\text{Se} - z_{\alpha/2}\text{SE}(\text{Se}), \quad \text{Se} + z_{\alpha/2}\text{SE}(\text{Se})\right)$$ (7.6)

where $Z_{\alpha/2}$ is the $100(1-\alpha/2)$th percentile of a standard normal distribution (usually α is 0.05).

Example 7.1 Cervical cancer screening research was carried out in Shanxi province in rural China in 2007, involving 2388 women aged 30–54 years [8]. All women were assessed by the Digene High-Risk HPV HC2 DNA Test (HC2), and 70 women had CIN2+ (moderate or severe cervical intraepithelial neoplasia or cancer). The results of the test with 1.0 as the cutoff value for HC2 test are shown in Table 7.3.

We have

$$\mathrm{Se} = \frac{68}{70} \times 100\ \% = 97.1\ \%, \quad \mathrm{SE}\left(\mathrm{Se}\right) = \sqrt{\frac{68 \times 2}{\left(68+2\right)^3}} = 2.0\ \%$$

95 % CI of Se:

$$\left(97.1\ \% - 1.96 \times 2.0\ \%,\ 97.1\ \% + 1.96 \times 2.0\ \%\right) = \left(93.2\ \%,\ 100\ \%\right)$$

$$\mathrm{Sp} = \frac{1985}{2318} \times 100\ \% = 85.6\ \%, \quad \mathrm{SE}\left(\mathrm{Sp}\right) = \sqrt{\frac{333 \times 1985}{\left(333+1985\right)^3}} = 0.7\ \%$$

95 % CI of Sp:

$$\left(85.6\ \% - 1.96 \times 0.7\ \%,\ 85.6\ \% + 1.96 \times 0.7\ \%\right) = \left(84.2\ \%,\ 87.1\ \%\right).$$

Similarly, FPR and FNR can be obtained simultaneously:

$$\mathrm{FPR} = \frac{333}{2318} \times 100\ \% = 14.4\ \%,$$

and

$$\mathrm{FNR} = \frac{2}{70} \times 100\ \% = 2.9\ \%.$$

In this study, both Se and Sp were relatively high, and FNR was low, all of which indicated a good performance of HC2 test itself.

Table 7.3 Results of HC2 screening test for CIN2+

	CIN2+		
HC2 test	Present	Absent	Total
Positive	68	333	401
Negative	2	1985	1987
Total	70	2318	2388

Joint Test

One usual way to increase the sensitivity and specificity of a test is to use multiple or repeat tests in "parallel" or in "series." In parallel testing, when any of tests is positive, the diagnosis is judged as positive. Otherwise, it is judged as negative. In a series of tests, a positive result can be obtained only when all tests are positive. The parallel test improves the sensitivity but lowers the specificity, while the series test improves the specificity but lowers the sensitivity.

Example 7.2 In the example above, the women were also assessed by liquid-based cytology test (LBC), and 68 were eventually diagnosed as CIN2+.

From the results of joint testing of LBC and HC2 for CIN2+ screening (Table 7.4), we can see the influence of joint testing on Se and Sp (Table 7.5).

The parallel test of LBC and HC2 increased the sensitivity from 97.1 to 98.5 % and decreased the specificity from 86.0 to 85.8 %. The series test reduced the sensitivity from 97.1 to 83.8 % and increased the specificity from 86.0 to 97.1 %. Thus, the choice of parallel or series tests should depend on the objective of the research.

Table 7.4 Results of joint screening test for CIN2+

Results of tests		CIN2+		
LBC	HC2	Present	Absent	Total
Positive	Negative	1	4	5
Negative	Positive	9	253	262
Positive	Positive	57	65	122
Negative	Negative	1	1948	1949
Total		68	2270	2338

Table 7.5 Estimates of Se and Sp of joint testing for LBC and HC2

Tests	Se	Sp
LBC	58/68 = 85.3 %	2201/2270 = 97.0 %
HC2	66/68 = 97.1 %	1952/2270 = 86.0 %
Parallel	67/68 = 98.5 %	1948/2270 = 85.8 %
Series	57/68 = 83.8 %	2205/2270 = 97.1 %

Combined Measures of Sensitivity and Specificity

When comparing the validity of two or more diagnostic tests, it is often difficult to determine which test is superior because both sensitivity and specificity must be accounted for. Several indicators combining measures of sensitivity and specificity are recommended in practice, such as accuracy, likelihood ratio (LR), and Youden's Index.

Accuracy of the test: the proportion of all tests that are correct classifications.

$$\text{Accuracy} = \frac{a+d}{a+b+c+d} \times 100 \ \% \tag{7.7}$$

The likelihood ratio for a positive test (LR+) and the likelihood ratio for a negative test (LR−), respectively.

$$\text{LR}+ = \frac{\text{Se}}{(1-\text{Sp})}, \quad \text{LR}- = \frac{(1-\text{Se})}{\text{Sp}} \tag{7.8}$$

For $\text{LR}+s$ greater than 1, the greater the value, the better the validity of the diagnostic test. While for $\text{LR}-s$ less than 1, the smaller value indicates better validity.

$$\text{Youden's Index} = \text{Se} + \text{Sp} - 1 \tag{7.9}$$

Youden's Index value between 0 and 1, and the greater the Youden's Index, the better the validity of the diagnostic test.

Example 7.1 (continued) Using the data in Table 7.3, we have the following results:

$$\text{Accuracy} = \frac{68+1985}{2388} \times 100 \ \% = 86.0 \ \%$$

$$\text{LR} + = \frac{97.1 \ \%}{1 - 85.6 \ \%} = 6.74, \quad \text{LR} - = \frac{1 - 97.1 \ \%}{85.6 \ \%} = 0.03$$

Youden's Index $= 97.1 \ \% + 85.6 \ \% - 1 = 0.83$.

Results of above four combined measures indicated that the validity of the test was relatively high.

Positive and Negative Predictive Value

Sensitivity and specificity are properties of a test itself and are only used to decide whether the test can be used. However, in practice, clinicians are more concerned with the chance of having the disease given a test's results. Two types of predictive values (positive and negative) are widely used to answer this question.

Positive-predictive value (PPV) is the probability of disease in a patient given a positive (abnormal) test result:

$$PPV = \frac{Se \times Prevalence}{Se \times Prevalence + (1 - Sp) \times (1 - Prevalence)} \qquad (7.10)$$

Negative-predictive value (NPV) is the probability of no disease given a negative (normal) test result:

$$NPV = \frac{Sp \times (1 - Prevalence)}{Sp \times (1 - Prevalence) + (1 - Se) \times Prevalence} \qquad (7.11)$$

The predictive values of test results were determined by sensitivity, specificity, and disease prevalence, while prevalence of the disease plays a very important role in calculating PPV and NPV. Under the condition that the testing population is a representative random sample of the source population, the above two formulae can be simplified as [9]:

$$PPV = \frac{a}{a+b} \times 100~\%, \quad NPV = \frac{d}{c+d} \times 100~\% \qquad (7.12)$$

Example 7.1 (continued) Based on the data in Table 7.3, the calculation of PPV and NPV for a random sample are:

$$PPV = \frac{68}{401} \times 100~\% = 17.0~\%, \quad NPV = \frac{1985}{1987} \times 100~\% = 99.9~\%$$

The result of PPV indicated only 17 % patients with abnormal HC2 had CIN2+, while 99.9 % of NPV results indicated a person with a normal HC2 almost free from CIN2+.

The low PPV in this study is due to a relative low prevalence of CIN2+ ($(68+2)/2388 = 0.029$). However, the NPV was almost 100 %, and both the sensitivity and the specificity are high, which indicated that the diagnostic value of cervical-cancer screening is quite high.

Receiver Operating Characteristic Curve

When test results extend from binary to ranked or continuous response, sensitivity and specificity can vary with different positive standards. Table 7.6 shows results of sensitivity and specificity with different cutoff values selected.

From Table 7.6, when the cutoff values of HC2 increased from 0.0 to 2500.0 (pg/mL), the Se decreased from 100.0 to 0.0 %; correspondingly, Sp increased from 0.0 to 100.0 % meanwhile. However, problems arise on how to comprehensively measure the validity of a test and how to ascertain an optimal cutoff value. The receiver operating characteristic (ROC) curve is a suitable method in this situation.

Table 7.6 Estimates for Se and Sp of different cutoff values of the HC2 test

Level of HC2 (pg/mL)	Se (%)	Sp (%)
0.0	100.0	0.0
0.2	100.0	31.8
0.5	98.6	82.6
1.0	97.1	85.6
2.0	95.7	87.8
10.0	87.1	90.5
20.0	82.9	92.3
50.0	72.9	94.4
200.0	55.7	97.2
1000.0	17.1	99.4
2500.0	0.0	100.0

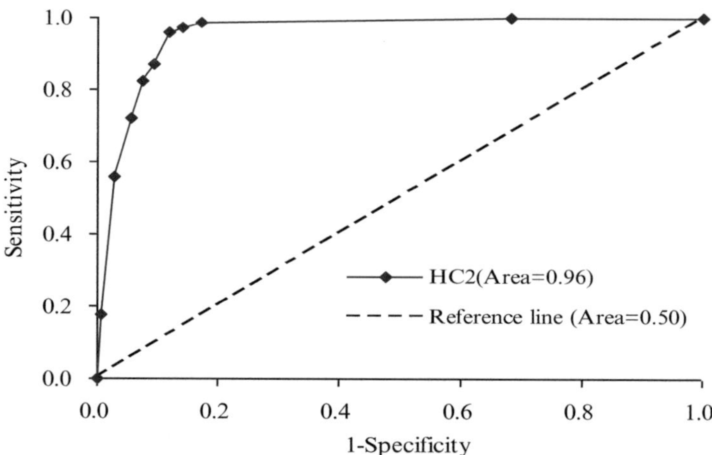

Fig. 7.4 Receiver operating characteristic curve for the HC2 test

The ROC curve was developed in the 1950s for evaluating radar signals detection. Only recently have they become commonly applied in healthcare [10, 11]. ROC curves can be presented by plotting sensitivity on the Y-axis against $1 -$ specificity on the X-axis. For example, Fig. 7.4 presents a empirical ROC curve for the HC2 test, using data from Table 7.6.

Interpretation of the ROC Curve

The solid line in Fig. 7.4 represents the performance of the HC2 test, on which each point corresponds to the values of sensitivity and $1 -$ specificity given a certain cutoff value. The dashed straight line from the bottom left corner to the top right corner, termed the diagnostic reference line, represents the performance of a hypothetical test that is completely useless. In practice, there is virtually always some overlap of the values in the two groups, so the curve will lie somewhere between these extremes.

Area Under the ROC Curve

The area under the ROC curve (AUC) can be used for quantitatively assessing the validity of a test. This area can be interpreted as the probability that a random person with a disease has a higher value of the measure than a random person without the disease. A test would yield a value of area under the curve in the range 0.5–1.0, with higher value corresponding to higher diagnostic power. In Table 7.6, for example, the HC2 test yields an area under the curve of 0.96 ($p < 0.001$), indicating that the HC2 test is of high value in the screening test of cervical cancer.

Selection of the Cutoff Value

How is the cutoff value selected when a test is demonstrated to be effective? As a general rule, cutoff values in the upper left-hand region of a ROC curve represent a reasonable trade-off between test sensitivity and specificity. In the example of HC2 test, the cutoff value 2.0 of HC2 on the graph represents a reasonable choice with a sensitivity of 95.7 % and specificity of 87.8 % compared to other cutoff values.

The selection of a specific cutoff value also depends on the intended use of the test. Usually, high specificity may be desired for a mass screening test to avoid overburdening the health service. While, in a screening test for cancer, it would be desirable to have a test of high sensitivity (and few false negatives), since failure to detect this condition early is often fatal. In Example 7.1, an HC2 cutoff level in the 0.5–2.5 (pg/mL) range seems to be best for balancing sensitivity and specificity. Thus, a cut-off value of 1.0 was selected in this study.

Comparison of Area Under the ROC Curves

Another important application of the ROC curves is to compare different tests synthetically. For Example 7.2, the ROC curve for the HC2 test could be compared with the ROC curve for the LBC test. The result indicated that, although the plots (Fig. 7.5) show that both HC2 and LBC are statistically significant compared with reference line ($p < 0.001$), they were not significantly different from each other ($p > 0.05$).

The main advantages of the ROC curve are: (1) simple and intuitive, i.e., clinical validity can be observed graphically; and, (2) it is not affected by the prevalence of disease in the test population.

In summary, a screening or diagnostic test can be influenced by many factors derived from the diagnostic method itself, as well as human behavior or environmental conditions. However, rational application of a clinical diagnostic test cannot occur without the proper evaluation of the test.

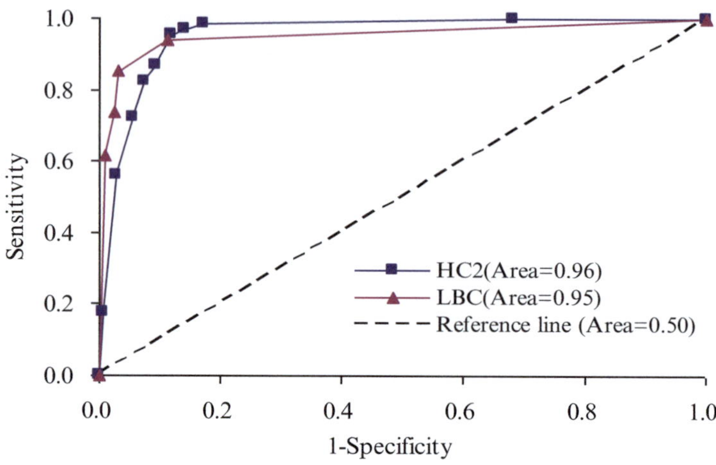

Fig. 7.5 Empirical ROC curves for the HC2 test and LBC test

Statistical Methods for Cancer Etiology Research

Compared with other non-communicable diseases, malignant tumors occur very rarely in the population. Case–control studies provide a relatively simple and fast way to investigate risk factors for a rare disease and play an important role in cancer epidemiological research.

Case–Control Study Design and Odds Ratio Estimation

A case–control study design (see Fig. 7.6) begins with the disease and looks backward to prior exposures. The investigators enroll cases and controls that are a representative of the source population from which the cases come, collect data on disease occurrence at one point and exposures at a previous point, and then explore the differences in exposure between cases and controls.

Figure 7.6 can be represented as a 2×2 contingency table, Table 7.7 below:

Odds Ratio Estimation

The odds ratio (OR) is the main effect measure for the association between exposure and disease in a case–control study, and it indicates the strength or magnitude of association between a disease and an exposure. The estimate for OR can be given by

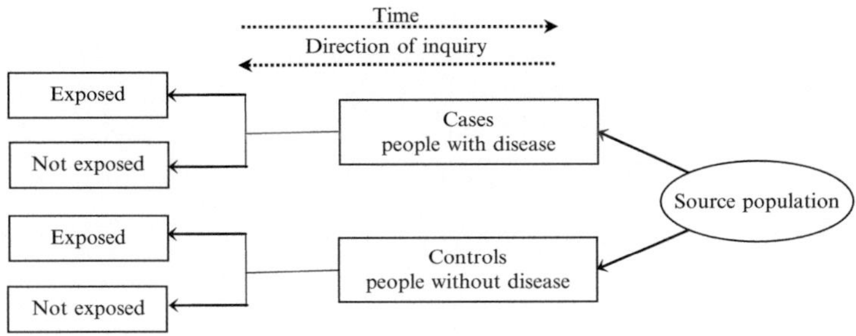

Fig. 7.6 Case–control study design

Table 7.7 Frequency distribution of cases and controls according to exposure

Diseases	Exposure		Total
	Yes	No	
Yes	a	b	$a+b$
No	c	d	$c+d$
Total	$a+c$	$b+d$	$a+b+c+d=n$

$$\widehat{OR} = \frac{\left[a/(a+b)\right]/\left[b/(a+b)\right]}{\left[c/(c+d)\right]/\left[d/(c+d)\right]} = \frac{a/b}{c/d} = \frac{ad}{bc} \tag{7.13}$$

$\ln(\widehat{OR})$, is the logarithmic transformation of $\widehat{OR}$ and has an approximate normal distribution. The maximum likelihood estimate of variance $\ln\left(\widehat{OR}\right)$ is

$$\mathrm{Var}\left(\ln\left(\widehat{OR}\right)\right) = \frac{1}{a} + \frac{1}{b} + \frac{1}{c} + \frac{1}{d} \tag{7.14}$$

The $100(1-\alpha)\%$ (α is usually 0.05) CI for $\widehat{OR}$ is

$$\exp\left(\ln\left(\widehat{OR}\right) \pm Z_{\alpha/2}\sqrt{\frac{1}{a} + \frac{1}{b} + \frac{1}{c} + \frac{1}{d}}\right) \tag{7.15}$$

$Z_{\alpha/2}$ reflects the desired level of confidence (e.g., 95 % when $\alpha=0.05$). If the 95 % CI of OR does not include 1, it leads to the rejection of the null hypothesis (H_0: OR = 1), indicating the exposure is associated with disease (α =0.05).

Example 7.3 To explore the association between smoking and lung cancer death, a large-scale population-based case–control study was conducted during 1989–1991 in China. 35,407 lung cancer cases and 88,760 controls aged ≥ 35 years were investigated [12]. Data are presented in Table 7.8.

Table 7.8 Frequency distribution of lung cancer cases and controls according to smoking status

Lung cancer	Smoking		Total
	Yes	No	
Yes	28,364	7043	35,407
No	54,176	34,584	88,760
Total	82,540	41,627	124,167

The estimated OR for lung cancer death in smokers relative to nonsmokers was

$$\widehat{OR} = \frac{28,364 \times 34,584}{7043 \times 54,176} = 2.57$$

The 95 % CI for OR was

$$\exp\left(\ln 2.57 \pm 1.96 \sqrt{\frac{1}{28,364} + \frac{1}{7043} + \frac{1}{54,176} + \frac{1}{34,584}} \right) = (2.50, 2.65)$$

The lower boundary of the 95 % CI for OR is greater than 1. We have significant evidence ($\alpha = 0.05$) that smoking is associated with lung cancer death. The risk of lung cancer death for a smoker was 2.57 times higher than that for a nonsmoker.

Stratification Analysis

In a case–control study, the association of disease and exposure can be distorted by other factors (confounders), so it is necessary to apply some other methods to identify and adjust for confounding. Stratified analysis is the usual method to control for confounding during data analysis. The Cochran–Mantel–Haenszel (CMH) method (1959) is commonly used for stratified adjustment of OR in case–control study. Suppose a confounder has h stratum, the data can be tabulated as h 2×2 tables (Table 7.9).

The CMH formula allows calculation of an overall, unconfounded, and adjusted effect estimate of a given exposure for a specific disease by combining (pooling) stratum-specific OR_i ($i = 1, 2, \ldots, h$). The estimate of OR_{cmh} is computed as

Table 7.9 Frequency distribution of cases and controls according to exposure in each stratum

Strata 1				...	Strata h			
	Exposure					Exposure		
Disease	Yes	No	Total	...	Disease	Yes	No	Total
Yes	a_1	b_1	a_1+b_1	...	Yes	a_h	b_h	a_h+b_h
No	c_1	d_1	c_1+d_1		No	c_h	d_h	c_h+d_h
Total	a_1+c_1	b_1+d_1	$a_1+b_1+c_1+d_1=n_1$	...	Total	a_h+c_h	b_h+d_h	$a_h+b_h+c_h+d_h=n_h$

$$\widehat{\mathrm{OR}}_{\mathrm{cmh}} = \frac{\sum_{i=1}^{h} a_i d_i / n_i}{\sum_{i=1}^{h} b_i c_i / n_i} \tag{7.16}$$

The Robins–Breslow–Greenland (RBG) estimate of $\mathrm{Var}\left(\ln\left(\widehat{\mathrm{OR}}_{\mathrm{cmh}}\right)\right)$ is

$$\mathrm{Var}\left(\ln\left(\widehat{\mathrm{OR}}_{\mathrm{cmh}}\right)\right) = \frac{\sum_{i=1}^{h}(a_i+d_i)a_i d_i/n_i^2}{2\left(\sum_{i=1}^{h} a_i d_i/n_i\right)^2} + \frac{\sum_{i=1}^{h}\left[(a_i+d_i)a_i d_i + (b_i+c_i)b_i c_i\right]/n_i^2}{2\left(\sum_{i=1}^{h} a_i d_i/n_i\right)\left(\sum_{i=1}^{h} b_i c_i/n_i\right)}$$

$$+ \frac{\sum_{i=1}^{h}(b_i+c_i)b_i c_i/n_i^2}{2\left(\sum_{i=1}^{h} b_i c_i/n_i\right)^2} \tag{7.17}$$

The 95 % CI for $\mathrm{OR}_{\mathrm{cmh}}$ is

$$\exp\left(\ln\left(\widehat{\mathrm{OR}}_{\mathrm{cmh}}\right) \pm 1.96\sqrt{\mathrm{Var}\left(\ln\left(\widehat{\mathrm{OR}}_{\mathrm{cmh}}\right)\right)}\right) \tag{7.18}$$

Similarly, if the 95 % CI does not include 1, we reject null hypothesis (H_0:$\mathrm{OR}_{\mathrm{cmh}}=1$), that is, the disease is significantly associated with the exposure ($\alpha = 0.05$) after adjusting for the effect of the confounder by stratification analysis.

The assumption of the CMH method is the homogeneity in the stratum-specific OR_i. If the assumption is not satisfied, this indicates that there is interaction between the stratification factor and exposure, then we should report stratum-specific OR_i separately and also fit regression model to identify and estimate the interaction.

Following Example 7.3, we can consider that the association between smoking and lung cancer deaths may be confounded by area (categorized into urban and rural areas). Next, we compute the area-adjusted OR for lung cancer deaths in smokers relative to nonsmokers. The data from Table 7.8 were divided into two 2×2 contingency tables displayed as Table 7.10.

Table 7.10 Frequency distribution of lung cancer cases and controls according to area and smoking status

Urban area				Rural area			
	Smoking					Smoking	
Lung cancer	Yes	No	Total	Lung cancer	Yes	No	Total
Yes	23,777	6052	29,829	Yes	4587	991	5578
No	33,491	23,907	57,398	No	20,685	10,677	31,362
Total	57,268	29,959	87,227	Total	25,272	11,668	36,940

The estimated OR adjusted by area is

$$\widehat{OR}_{cmh} = \frac{\sum (a_i d_i / n_i)}{\sum (b_i c_i / n_i)}$$
$$= \frac{23,777 \times 23,907 / 87,227 + 4587 \times 10,677 / 36,940}{33,491 \times 6052 / 87,227 + 20,685 \times 991 / 36,940}$$
$$= \frac{7842.56}{2878.60} = 2.72$$

The variance of $\ln\left(\widehat{OR}_{cmh}\right)$ is

$$Var\left(\ln\left(\widehat{OR}_{cmh}\right)\right) = 0.000232$$

The 95 % CI for OR_{cmh} is

$$\exp\left(\ln 2.72 \pm 1.96 \times \sqrt{0.000232}\right) = (2.64, 2.81)$$

The 95 % CI does not include 1, which indicates that the association between smoking and lung cancer deaths was statistically significant after adjustment for area ($\alpha = 0.05$). The area-adjusted risk of lung cancer death for a smoker is 2.72 times higher than that for a nonsmoker. The area-adjusted OR (2.72) is different from the crude OR (2.57), which indicates that area is a confounder for the association between smoking and lung cancer death.

Although the CMH method is a simple and commonly used way to control confounders, it has two important limitations: (1) if there is more than one single confounder, the application of this formula is laborious because of the greater number of strata and demands a relatively large sample size; and, (2) this method requires continuous confounders to be constrained into a limited number of categories, and potentially generating residual confounding. Thus, if we need to control several confounders or continuous confounders and quantify the interaction between factors, logistic regression can be used as it has superiority over stratification analysis in these aspects.

Application of the Logistic Regression Model

We define the binary outcome variable Y ($Y=1$ if a disease is present, otherwise $Y=0$) with probabilities $\Pr(Y=1)=\pi$ and $\Pr(Y=0)=1-\pi$, which follows Bernoulli distribution $B(\pi)$. If there are n such random variables Y_1, Y_2, ..., Y_n, which are independent with $\Pr(Y_i=1)=\pi_i$, then their joint probability is

$$\prod_{i=1}^{n}\pi_i^{y_i}\left(1-\pi_i\right)^{1-y_i}=\exp\left[\sum_{i=1}^{n}\left(y_i\ln\left(\frac{\pi_i}{1-\pi_i}\right)+\ln\left(1-\pi_i\right)\right)\right] \qquad (7.19)$$

We model the probability π_i as

$$g\left(\pi_i\right)=X_i^T\beta \qquad (7.20)$$

where $X_i=\left(X_{i1},X_{i2},\ldots,X_{ik}\right)$ is a vector of explanatory variables, β is a vector of parameters and $g(.)$ is a link function, π_i and $X_i^T\beta$ are restricted to the interval $[0, 1]$ and $\left(-\infty, +\infty\right)$ respectively. Different link functions will create different models. If we choose logistic link function, we could get a logistic regression model as follows

$$\ln\left(\frac{\pi_i}{1-\pi_i}\right)=\beta_0+\sum_{j=1}^{k}\beta_j X_{ij} \qquad (7.21)$$

where $\ln\left[\pi_i/\left(1-\pi_i\right)\right]$ is expressed as a linear function of exposures X_i. β_j denotes the average increase of $\ln\left[\pi_i/\left(1-\pi_i\right)\right]$ for 1 unit increase in X_{ij}. An important interpretation of the logistic regression model in epidemiologic studies uses the odds and the odds ratio. The odds of response equals 1 (i.e., the odds of a disease) is

$$\frac{\pi_i}{1-\pi_i}=\exp\left(\beta_0+\sum_{j=1}^{k}\beta_j X_{ij}\right) \qquad (7.22)$$
$$=\exp\left(\beta_0\right)\exp\left(\beta_1 X_{i1}\right)\exp\left(\beta_1 X_{i2}\right)\ldots\exp\left(\beta_k X_{ik}\right)$$

This exponential relationship provides an interpretation for β_j, the odds multiply by $\exp(\beta_j)$ for 1 unit increase in X_{ij}. That is, the odds at level $X_{ij}+1$ equal the odds at X_{ij} multiplied by $\exp(\beta_j)$. The odds ratio of disease for people with $X_{ij}+1$ relative to people with X_{ij} adjusting the effect of other covariates is

$$\text{OR}=\frac{\exp\left[\beta_0+\beta_1 X_{i1}+\beta_2 X_{i2}+\cdots+\beta_j\left(X_{ij}+1\right)+\cdots+\beta_k X_{ik}\right]}{\exp\left[\beta_0+\beta_1 X_{i1}+\beta_2 X_{i2}+\cdots+\beta_j X_{ij}+\cdots+\beta_k X_{ik}\right]}$$
$$=\exp\left[\beta_j\left(X_{ij}+1-X_{ij}\right)\right] \qquad (7.23)$$
$$=\exp\left(\beta_j\right)$$

The estimation of OR is $\exp(\hat{\beta}_j)$ and the 95 % CI for OR is

$$\exp\left[\hat{\beta}_j \pm 1.96 \; \mathrm{SE}\left(\hat{\beta}_j\right)\right] \tag{7.24}$$

Once we have fit a particular multiple logistic regression model, we should test the significance of global model and specific coefficient and test the goodness of fit: (1) the likelihood ratio test and Wald test are usually used for the global model test and specific coefficient test. The Wald test is adequate for large samples, the likelihood-ratio test is more powerful and more reliable for sample sizes and often used in practice; (2) the goodness of fit test is to measure the difference between the observed and fitted value. The deviation test, Pearson test, and Hosmer–Lemeshow tests are usually used. Deviation and Pearson tests require sufficient replication within the subgroups. If the data are sparse, Hosmer–Lemeshow test is much more reliable.

The logistic regression modeling strategy generally involves three stages: Variable specification is addressed first. This step allows the investigator to confirm clinically or biologically meaningful variables of interest based on specialized knowledge. An interaction assessment is carried out next, prior to the assessment of confounding. If there is strong evidence of interaction involving certain variables, then the assessment of confounding involving these variables becomes irrelevant. The final stage of strategy calls for the assessment of confounding followed by consideration of precision. This means that it is more important to obtain a valid point estimate of the exposure–disease relationship that controls for confounding than to get a narrow confidence interval around a biased estimate that does not control for confounding.

Following Example 7.3, although the CMH method can compute the area-adjusted OR of lung cancer deaths for smokers relative to nonsmokers, we want to apply a logistic regression model to control the effect of area and age simultaneously and try to explore the interaction among them. The logistic regression modeling strategy is as follows: (1) smoking is the variable of interest—we try to explore the interaction between certain variables, and to ascertain that there is an interaction between smoking and area; and, (2) we continue to control the effect of age which is a continuous confounder for the association between smoking and lung cancer death. The final model is shown in Table 7.11.

The association between smoking and lung cancer death varies for different methods. The estimated ORs for different analyses are shown in Table 7.12.

This table shows that the logistic regression model has controlled for the effect of age and area simultaneously and identified the interaction between area and smoking, so we have reason to believe that the result adjusted by the logistic regression

Table 7.11 Results of logistic regression model

Variables	DF	$\hat{\beta}$	SE $(\hat{\beta})$	P	$\widehat{\mathrm{OR}}$	95 % CI for OR	
Smoking	1	0.87	0.0370	<0.0001	2.39	2.22	2.57
Area	1	1.00	0.0362	<0.0001	2.72	2.53	2.92
Age	1	0.0011	0.0005	0.0317	1.0011	1.0001	1.0022
Smoking* area	1	0.16	0.0406	<0.0001	1.18	1.09	1.27

*denotes multiple sign

Table 7.12 Estimated ORs of lung cancer death for smokers vs. nonsmokers based on different analyses

Analytic method	$\widehat{OR}$
Crude OR (ad/bc based on 2×2 contingency table)	2.57
Area stratification adjusted OR (CMH method)	2.72
Multi-variables adjusted OR (logistic regression model)	2.39

model was more reliable than the crude OR and that of stratification analysis. The risk of lung cancer death for smokers is 2.39 times higher than that of nonsmokers and the effect of interaction between smoking and area is 1.18, indicating that smoking could accelerate the risk of lung cancer deaths among urban smokers.

Statistical Methods for Cancer Prognosis Research

It is very important to identify the factors associated with cancer prognosis to help improve the survival rate and quality of life of cancer patients. Cancer prognosis research usually needs to follow up patients to collect exposure information and endpoints, so a cohort study is commonly used in such research.

Cohort Study Design

Cohort studies, also called follow-up studies, begin with a group of people who are free of disease and who are classified into subgroups according to exposure to a potential cause of disease or outcome (Fig. 7.7). Variables of interest are specified and measured, and the whole cohort is followed up over time to determine how the subsequent development of new cases of the disease differs between the groups with and without exposure.

Kaplan–Meier Method and Log-Rank Test

The assessment of cancer prognosis usually relies on time-to-event data, and non-compliant or lost to follow up are inevitable in this process, which is called censoring. Survival analysis is the common choice to analyze cancer prognosis data with censoring. In survival analysis, two functions are of major interest, namely the hazard function $h(t)$ and survival function $S(t)$. The $h(t)$ is the instantaneous event rate at time t for an individual surviving to time t. The $S(t)$ is the probability of surviving to time t. The relationship between the two functions can be expressed as $S(t) = \exp\left(-\int_0^t h(u)\,du\right)$. The Kaplan–Meier (KM) method (also known as the product-limit method) was widely used to describe the survival process and

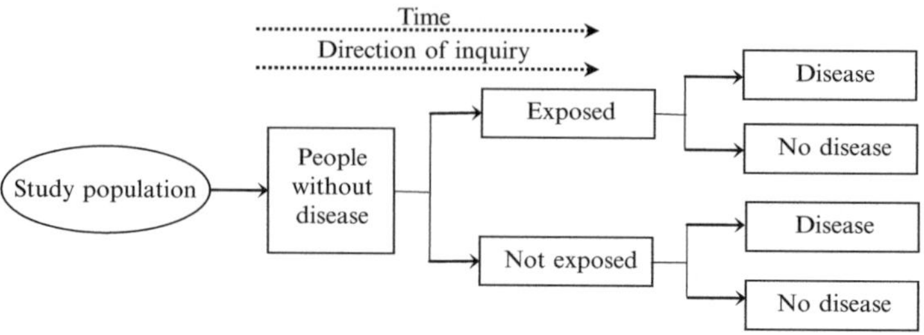

Fig. 7.7 Cohort study design

estimate $S(t)$. Suppose there are k distinct event times $t_1 < t_2 < \cdots < t_k$, and there are n_j individuals at the risk of an event at time t_j, for those who are censored at exactly t_j they are also considered to be at risk at t_j, let d_j individuals have events at time t_j. The $S(t)$ at t_j is estimated by the formula below:

$$\hat{S}\left(t_j\right) = \left(1 - \frac{d_1}{n_1}\right) \times \left(1 - \frac{d_2}{n_2}\right) \times \cdots \times \left(1 - \frac{d_j}{n_j}\right) \quad j = 1,\, 2,\dots,k \tag{7.25}$$

The variance of $\hat{S}(t_j)$ is estimated by Greenwood's formula given by

$$SE\left[\hat{S}\left(t_j\right)\right] = \hat{S}\left(t_j\right)\sqrt{\sum_{i=1}^{j}\frac{d_i}{n_i\left(n_i - d_i\right)}} \tag{7.26}$$

The 95 % CI for $S(t_j)$ can be approximately given by

$$\hat{S}\left(t_j\right) \pm 1.96SE\left[\hat{S}\left(t_j\right)\right] \tag{7.27}$$

Plotting a graph of survival rate against time produces a survival curve that can directly show the change in survival rate with time.

The effects of two treatments can be assessed by comparing survival rate at a specific time point or median survival time. However, we usually gain more information if we compare the $S(t)$ for all time points, the test hypothesis test for $\hat{S}_1(t)$ and $\hat{S}_2(t)$ is

$$H_0 : S_1\left(t\right) = S_2\left(t\right) \text{ for all } t \text{ vs. } H_1 : S_1\left(t\right) \neq S_2\left(t\right) \text{ for some } t.$$

The above hypothesis can be assessed by performing a log-rank test (1966) with the purpose of calculating the number of events expected for each group and comparing the expected number of events with the observed number of events in each group under the null hypothesis. The log-rank statistic can be computed by the following steps:

1. Pool the two groups and sort the event times in ascending order. Suppose there are r distinct event times $t_1 < t_2 < \cdots < t_r$. At time t_j (j=1,2,...,r), we assume there are n_{1j}, n_{2j}, and n_j individuals at risk of the event and d_{1j}, d_{2j}, and d_j individuals who have had an event in groups 1, 2, and the two groups combined, respectively.
2. Calculate the expected number of events and its variance for each group, here we take group 1 as example, e_{1j} and $\mathrm{Var}(e_{1j})$ at time t_j can be given by

$$e_{1j} = n_{1j}d_j / n_j, \quad \mathrm{Var}\left(e_{1j}\right) = \frac{n_{1j}n_{2j}d_j\left(n_j - d_j\right)}{n_j^2\left(n_j - 1\right)}$$

3. Calculate the log-rank statistic which has a chi-square distribution with one degree of freedom using the following formula

$$\chi^2 = \frac{\left(\sum_{j=1}^{r}(d_{1j} - e_{1j})\right)^2}{\sum_{j=1}^{r}\mathrm{Var}\left(e_{1j}\right)}$$ (7.28)

For a given confidence level α (usually 0.05), if $\chi^2 > \chi^2_{\alpha,\,1}$ then we reject H_0, that is, the two survival curves are significant different. The conclusion will not change if the group 2 is used to calculate the statistics above.

Example 7.4 In a clinical prognostic study concerned with breast cancer, 74 breast cancer patients who had surgery were followed up for 10 years to assess the prognosis. Data were collected as follows: age at diagnosis (X_1: years), type of metastasis (X_2: 1 = multiple metastasis, 0 = single metastasis), hormone receptors (X_3: 1 = positive, 0 = negative), survival status (status: 1 = death, 0 = censored), and survival time (month). We consider comparing the survival experience between patients with single metastasis and patients with multiple metastasis.

The survival rate for the single metastasis group and multiple metastasis group was estimated (see Table 7.13).

Table 7.13 Survival times and rates by single metastasis and multiple metastasis groups

Group	No	Time t_j	Death d_j	Survival n_j	Survival probability $p_j = (n_j - d_j)/n_j$	Survival rate $\hat{S}(t_j)$	SE($\hat{S}(t_j)$)
Single	1	15	1	40	0.9750	0.9750	0.0247
	2	21	1	39	0.9744	0.9500	0.0345
	3	23	1	38	0.9737	0.9250	0.0416
	4	28	1	37	0.9730	0.9000	0.0474
	5	29	1	36	0.9722	0.8750	0.0523
	⋮	⋮	⋮	⋮	⋮	⋮	⋮
	34	130+	0	1	1.0000	0.1418	0.0879
Multiple	1	12	1	34	0.9706	0.9706	0.0290
	2	19	1	33	0.9697	0.9412	0.0404
	3	22+	0	32	1.0000	0.9412	0.0404
	4	23	2	31	0.9355	0.8805	0.0561
	5	24	1	29	0.9655	0.8501	0.0619
	⋮	⋮	⋮	⋮	⋮		⋮
	32	120	1	1	0.0000	0.0000	0.0616

+: denotes censoring

(continued)

Plotting the $S(t)$ against time, we can obtain two survival curves:

Figure 7.8 shows that the survival rate of the single metastasis group at each time period was higher than that of the multiple metastasis group. We use the log-rank test to compare the two curves, the expected number of events and its variance for the two groups at time t_j was seen in Table 7.14.

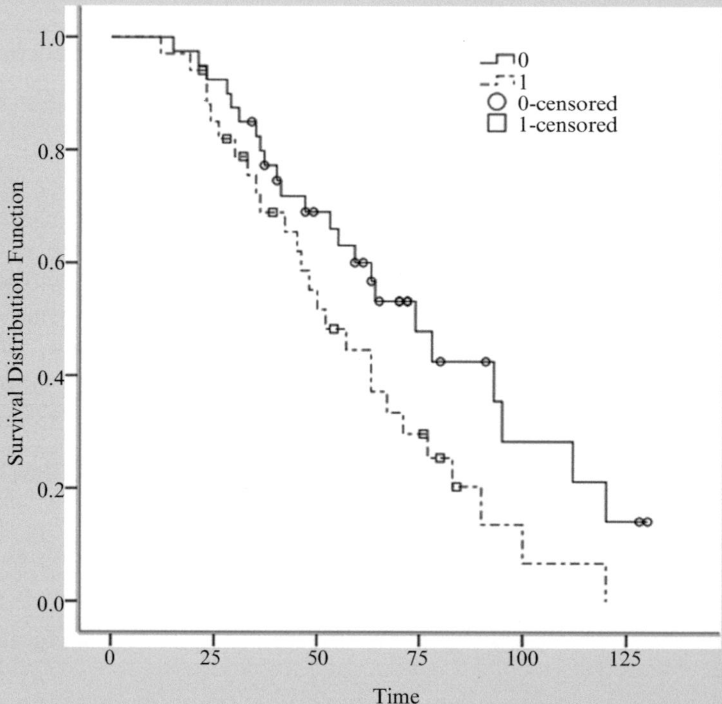

Fig. 7.8 Survival curves of single metastasis and multiple metastasis groups

Table 7.14 Expected number of events and its variance in the two groups

No	Time t_j	Single metastasis group				Multiple metastasis group				Total	
		n_{1j}	d_{1j}	e_{1j}	Var(e_{1j})	n_{2j}	d_{2j}	e_{2j}	Var(e_{2j})	n_j	d_j
1	12	40	0	0.5405	0.2484	34	1	0.4595	0.2484	74	1
2	15	40	1	0.5479	0.2477	33	0	0.4521	0.2477	73	1
3	19	39	0	0.5417	0.2483	33	1	0.4583	0.2483	72	1
4	21	39	1	0.5493	0.2476	32	0	0.4507	0.2476	71	1
5	22+	38	0	0.0000	0.0000	32	0	0.0000	0.0000	70	0
⋮	⋮	⋮	⋮	⋮	⋮	⋮	⋮	⋮	⋮	⋮	⋮
58	130+	1	0	0.0000	–	0	0	0.0000	–	1	0
Total			23	29.6154	11.3324		26	20.6154	11.3324	–	–

(continued)

The log-rank statistic based on one of the two groups (say, single metastasis group) was as follows:

$$\chi^2 = \frac{\left(\sum_{j=1}^{r}(d_{1j}-e_{1j})\right)^2}{\sum_{j=1}^{r}\mathrm{Var}\left(e_{1j}\right)} = \frac{\left(\sum_{j=1}^{r}d_{1j}-\sum_{j=1}^{r}e_{1j}\right)^2}{\sum_{j=1}^{r}\mathrm{Var}\left(e_{1j}\right)} = \frac{(23-29.6154)^2}{11.3324} = 3.8618$$

For a significance level 0.05, $\chi^2 > \chi^2_{0.05,\,1}$, which indicates that the two survival curves are different significantly. The single metastasis group has a higher survival rate than that of the multiple metastasis group.

Although the log-rank test is a popular method for comparing survival curves, it has three major limitations: (1) it is more likely to detect a difference between groups when the survival curves do not cross; (2) it can be used to compare survival curves with controlling for covariates with a little few stratum. However, if we want to control for continuous covariates or covariates with several stratum, the log-rank test does not work; (3) it does not provide a direct estimate of the magnitude of effect for one group relative to another group. All of these limitations can be overcomed by the application of a hazards regression model, such as the Cox proportional hazards model, which would be introduced in the following section.

Application of the Cox Proportional Hazards Model

The Cox proportional hazards model (1972) relates the hazard function to a number of covariates as follows:

$$h(t) = h_0(t)\exp\left(\beta_1 X_1 + \beta_2 X_2 + \cdots + \beta_k X_k\right) \tag{7.29}$$

where X_1, X_2, …,X_k are a collection of covariates, and $h_0(t)$ is an arbitrary and unspecified baseline hazard at time t, which represents the hazard for a person with the value 0 for all the covariates and can take any form, whereas in the parametric perspective it represents a specific distributional function. $\beta_j\,(j=1,\,2,\,…,k)$ represents the regression coefficient, which provides the effects of variable X_j on the hazard rate. Exponentiation of β_j generates the hazard ratio (HR) of variable X_j, which denotes the ratio of $h(t)$ for people with X_j+1 and people with X_j adjusting the effect of other covariates, and is given by

Table 7.15 Results of Cox regression model

Variables	DF	$\hat{\beta}$	SE($\hat{\beta}$)	P	$\widehat{HR}$	95 % CI for HR	
Type of metastasis	1	0.64	0.2950	0.0305	1.89	1.06	3.38
Hormone receptors	1	−0.42	0.3027	0.1687	0.66	0.36	1.19
Age	1	0.01	0.0171	0.3864	1.02	0.98	1.05

$$\text{HR} = \frac{h_0(t)\exp\left[\beta_1 X_1 + \cdots + \beta_j\left(X_j + 1\right) + \cdots + \beta_k X_k\right]}{h_0(t)\exp\left[\beta_1 X_1 + \cdots + \beta_j X_j + \cdots + \beta_k X_k\right]}$$
$$= \exp\left[\beta_j\left(X_j + 1 - X_j\right)\right] \tag{7.30}$$
$$= \exp\left(\beta_j\right)$$

The estimation of HR is $\exp(\hat{\beta}_j)$ and the 95 % CI for HR is

$$\exp\left[\hat{\beta}_j \pm 1.96\text{SE}\left(\hat{\beta}_j\right)\right] \tag{7.31}$$

As for the model assessment, the likelihood ratio test and Wald test are usually used for the global model test and specific coefficient test in Cox model, and we could use residuals (for example, martingale residual, deviance residual, score residual, and Schoenfeld residual) to examine the model adequacy.

Note that the Cox proportional hazards model is dependent on a proportional hazards assumption, which means that the hazard for one individual is proportional to the hazard for any other individual, and the proportionality constant is dependent on covariate values but independent of time. There is an overview of three methods for checking the assumption, that is, graphical approach, goodness of fit test based on Schoenfeld residuals and time-dependent variable test by adding a time-dependent interaction term $(X_j \times t)$ into the Cox model, and testing for statistical significance.

Following Example 7.4, we compared the survival curves of multiple metastasis and single metastasis groups above. Now we need to explore the prognostic factors that influence the survival rate of patients after surgery for breast cancer. A Cox model was applied and the results are presented in Table 7.15.

Table 7.15 shows that only the type of metastasis is statistically significant in the model. Patients with multiple metastasis would have worse prognosis, with a hazards rate 1.89 times higher than that of the single metastasis group. Age and hormone receptors were not statistically significant, but we think the two factors do have an influence based on specialized knowledge. So we would still adjust for age and hormone receptors and include them in the model.

Statistical Methods for Cancer Registration Data

In this section, we will introduce the common statistical methods for analysis of population-based cancer registration data, to help maximize the usefulness of the data collected through the adoption of uniform methods in cancer registration, especially in countries where the incidence and characteristics of the disease are poorly described.

Statistical analysis of cancer registry data is basically divided into three parts: (1) presentation of the basic results of the statistical report; (2) survival analysis; and, (3) application of statistical models. Because the method of survival analysis is the same as that in clinical research (as detailed in section "Statistical Methods for Cancer Prognosis Research"), we will mainly discuss part (1) because of its basic function in cancer registration and use a practical example of Poisson regression modeling to show how to carry out multivariate statistical analysis when data contain more information. Because the application of statistical models is broad and flexible, readers requiring more information may refer to related statistical books.

Presentation of the Basic Results of a Statistical Report

A key objective of a cancer registry is to produce statistics on the occurrence of cancer in a defined population. Population-based cancer registries in developing countries should be able to report their results in the same way as elsewhere. Cancer registry tables are usually divided into two sections: the statistics report and the analysis report, as partly presented in Table 7.16. The basic table is a frequency distribution of the number of cases during a specified time period according to cancer site, age, and sex. The distribution should be given by 5-year age groups

Table 7.16 Data on the incidence of lung cancer in 2007 (Cancer Registration in Beijing, China)

Age class	Male		Female	
	Cases	Incidence/100,000	Cases	Incidence/100,000
0–4	0	0.00	0	0.00
⋮	⋮	⋮	⋮	⋮
20–24	0	0.00	2	0.30
25–29	4	0.59	12	1.94
30–34	8	1.59	10	2.11
⋮	⋮	⋮	⋮	⋮
80–84	242	473.87	140	247.31
≥85	104	437.67	72	228.06
Crude rate	2515	67.35	1514	41.47
CUMI rate (aged 0–64)	1.74		0.93	
ASR China[a]	47.42		29.15	
ASR World[b]	37.36		25.32	
Truncated rate (aged 35–64)	44.67		26.12	

[a]Age-standard incidence rate per 100,000, China standard population in 2010
[b]World standard population in 2010

(e.g., 0–4, 5–9, 10–14, …, and $\geq$85 years, with A representing the number of groups ($A = 18$)); sometimes the 0–4 age group is further divided into two groups, i.e., 0 years old and 1–4 years old. If the table includes rates, the denominator on which they are based should be clearly stated. The common statistical indicators which are presented in a registry table are the crude rate, the age- and sex-specific incidence rate, and a summarizing set of rates, such as the standardized rate, cumulative rate, and shrinkage rate. The cancer incidence report represents the basic presentation of cancer registry data. It constitutes the key feedback report for physicians, health authorities, and the public on the occurrence of cancer.

Common Statistical Indicators in the Report

Incidence Rate

The incidence rate is a measure of the frequency with which an event, such as a new case of a cancer, occurs in the source population over a defined period of time. It is usually expressed, in the cancer registry report, as a rate per 100,000 person-years. The formula for calculating the incidence rate is as follows:

$$\text{Incidence rate} = \frac{\text{New cases occuring during a given time period}}{\text{Population at risk during the same time period}} \times 100,000 \quad (7.32)$$

Because the denominator of the incidence rate is person-year (its value may range from 0 to ∞), the rate is not interpretable as probability.

Incidence rates are of particular value in the study of disease etiology, since they provide information about the risk of developing a disease in different population groups. There have been many indices which have been developed to express disease occurrence in a community, such as:

Crude Incidence Rate

The crude (all-ages) rate per 100,000 person-years can be easily calculated by the formula:

$$\text{Crude rate} = \frac{R}{N} \times 100,000 \quad (7.33)$$

where R denotes the total number of new cases which have occurred in the source population, and N denotes the total person-years of observation.

Age-Specific Rate

When all cases are divided by known age, we may obtain an age-specific rate per 100,000 person-years denoted as a_i:

$$a_i = \frac{r_i}{n_i} \times 100,000 \quad (7.34)$$

where i denotes the age class, which is frequently divided into 18 groups ($A = 18$), r_i denotes the number of cases in the age class i, and n_i denotes the corresponding person-years of observation.

Cumulative Incidence Rate

The formula for calculating the cumulative incidence (CUMI) rate is as follows:

$$\text{CUMI rate} = \sum_{i=1}^{A} a_i t_i \tag{7.35}$$

where a_i denotes age-specific incidence rate, and t_i denotes the width of the age group.

The CUMI rate has important advantages as a method of reporting cancer incidence. It represents the probability that a person with no prior disease will develop the disease over a specified time period, and it dispenses with the rather arbitrary selection of the standard population, yet has the desired feature of summarizing the age-specific data.

In practice, however, it does not usually allow direct comparison of incidence rates between different countries because of differences in the age structure. For example, an older population may appear to have higher rates of certain cancers, not because of the presence of risk factors, but due to older age. This is a form of confounding. The so-called standardization is applied to reported rates to adjust for differences in age and possibly other confounders.

Age-Standardized Rate

There are two methods of age-standardization in widespread use, known as direct and indirect methods. We only introduce the direct method here since it has considerable interpretative advantages over the indirect method, and it is generally preferred whenever possible in cancer research.

The directly standardized (adjusted) rate consists of a weighted average of age-specific rates, where the weights reflect a known population structure. This structure is typically chosen as that of a country in a given census year, the so-called Standard Population. The age-standardized rate (ASR) is calculated from:

$$\text{ASR} = \frac{\sum a_i w_i}{\sum w_i} \tag{7.36}$$

where w_i is weight, which is the population present in the ith age class of the Standard Population, and a_i represents the age-specific rate in the ith age class.

It should be noted that many possible sets of weights (different standard populations) can be used. Use of different sets of weights will produce different values for the standardized rate. In cancer research, the most frequently used population is the World Standard Population (Table 7.17).

Table 7.17 World Standard Population of males in 2010

Age class index (i)	Age class	Population (w_i)	Age class index (i)	Age class	Population (w_i)
1.	0–4	9532	10.	45–49	5938
2.	5–9	9010	11.	50–54	5057
3.	10–14	8782	12.	55–59	4413
4.	15–19	8955	13.	60–64	3265
5.	20–24	9061	14.	65–69	2412
6.	25–29	8163	15.	70–74	1890
7.	30–34	7325	16.	75–79	1273
8.	35–39	7097	17.	80–84	740
9.	40–44	6664	18.	≥85	423
Total					100,000

Truncated Rate

The truncated age-standardized rate (TASR) can be written as follows:

$$\text{TASR} = \frac{\sum_{i=8}^{13} a_i w_i}{\sum_{i=8}^{13} w_i} \tag{7.37}$$

The calculation of rates is performed on the truncated age range of 35–64 years, mainly because of doubts about the accuracy of age-specific rates in the old populations, when diagnosis and recording of cancers may be much less certain.

Example 7.5 Calculation of lung cancer incidence rates per 100,000 person-years among Beijing men in 2007 (data from Table 7.16).

1. Crude incidence rate

$$\text{Crude rate} = \frac{R}{N} \times 100,000 = \frac{2515}{3,734,512} \times 100,000 = 67.35$$

2. Age-specified incidence rate at age 25–29 and at age ≥ 85 years

$$a_{25-29} = \frac{r_{25-29}}{n_{25-29}} \times 100,000 = \frac{4}{657,687} \times 100,000 = 0.59$$

$$a_{\geq 85} = \frac{r_{\geq 85}}{n_{\geq 85}} \times 100,000 = \frac{104}{23,801} \times 100,000 = 437.67$$

(continued)

3. Cumulative incidence rate (age 0–64 years)

$$\text{CUMI rate} = \sum_{i=1}^{13} a_i t_i = \left(0.59 + 1.59 + \cdots + 170.62\right) \times 5 = 1740.44$$

4. Age-standardized rate (ASR, World 2010)

$$\text{ASR} = \frac{\sum a_i w_i}{\sum w_i} = \frac{0.59 \times 8163 + \ldots + 437.67 \times 423}{100,000} = 37.36$$

5. Truncated rate (age 35–64 years)

$$\text{TASR} = \frac{\sum_{i=8}^{13} a_i w_i}{\sum_{i=8}^{13} w_i} = \frac{4.90 \times 7097 + \cdots + 170.62 \times 3265}{32,435} = 44.67$$

Comparison of Age-Standardized Rates

It is frequently of interest to compare the ASRs from different population groups, for example from two different geographical areas, ethnic groups, or from different time periods. The ratio between two ASRs, $\text{ASR}_1/\text{ASR}_2$ is called the standardized rate ratio (SRR) and represents the relative risk of disease in population 1 compared with population 2. It is usual to also calculate the statistical significance of the SRR (as an indication of whether the observed ratio is significantly different from unity). Several methods are available for calculating the exact CI of the SRR, but an approximation may be obtained with the following formula [13]:

$$\left(\frac{\text{ASR}_1}{\text{ASR}_2}\right)^{1 \pm \left(Z_{\alpha/2}/X\right)} \tag{7.38}$$

$$\text{where} \quad X = \frac{\text{ASR}_1 - \text{ASR}_2}{\sqrt{\text{SE}^2\left(\text{ASR}_1\right) + \text{SE}^2\left(\text{ASR}_2\right)}} \tag{7.39}$$

The standard error of ASR is

$$\text{SE}\left(\text{ASR}\right) = \frac{\sqrt{\sum \left[a_i w_i^2 \times \left(100,000 - a_i\right)/n_i\right]}}{\sum w_i} \tag{7.40}$$

Which is calculated based on the Poisson assumption for the age-specific rates [14], and $Z_{\alpha/2}$ reflects the desired level of confidence (e.g., 95 % when $\alpha = 0.05$).

Example 7.6 Comparison of ASR (World 2010) between men and women (Table 7.16).

The estimated SRR was $\mathrm{ASR}_1 / \mathrm{ASR}_2 = 37.36 / 25.32 = 1.48$, while $\mathrm{SE}(\mathrm{ASR}_1) = 0.0683$, $\mathrm{SE}(\mathrm{ASR}_2) = 0.0594$,

$$X = \frac{\mathrm{ASR}_1 - \mathrm{ASR}_2}{\sqrt{\mathrm{SE}^2(\mathrm{ASR}_1) + \mathrm{SE}^2(\mathrm{ASR}_2)}} = \frac{37.36 - 25.32}{\sqrt{(0.0683)^2 + (0.0594)^2}} = 133.03$$

Thus, the 95 % CI for $\mathrm{ASR}_1/\mathrm{ASR}_2$ is obtained as follows:

$$\left(1.48^{1-(1.96/133.03)}, 1.48^{1+(1.96/133.03)}\right) = (11.61,\ 12.49)$$

If the rates in the two populations were the same, the ratio $\mathrm{ASR}_1/\mathrm{ASR}_2$ would be 1. However, the estimated 95 % CI for this ratio (11.61, 12.49) does not contain this value, thus it can be concluded that the rates are significantly different at the 5 % level.

Testing for Trends in Age-Standardized Rates

As an extension to the testing of differences between pairs of ASRs described above, sometimes a set of ASRs are available for populations which are ordered according to some sort of scale. For example, for ASRs from different time periods. In this case, fitting a straight line regression equation is a common and suitable method of expressing a linear trend of cancer occurrence [13].

Linear regression equation—The equation of the linear relating Y to X is called the simple linear regression equation as given here:

$$Y = \alpha + \beta X + \varepsilon \tag{7.41}$$

where β is the slope of the line, $Y \sim N(\alpha + \beta X, \sigma^2)$, $\varepsilon \sim N(0, \sigma^2)$.

The estimate of the simple linear regression equation is given below:

$$\hat{Y} = a + bX \tag{7.42}$$

where $\hat{Y}$ is the expected value of Y for a given value of X; a and b are the least squares estimates of α and β, respectively, and are determined using the flowing equations:

$$b = \frac{\sum_{i=1}^{n}(x_i - \bar{x})(y_i - \bar{y})}{\sum_{i=1}^{n}(x_i - \bar{x})^2} = \frac{\sum_{i=1}^{n} x_i y_i - \dfrac{\left(\sum_{i=1}^{n} x_i\right)\left(\sum_{i=1}^{n} y_i\right)}{n}}{\sum_{i=1}^{n} x_i^2 - \dfrac{\left(\sum_{i=1}^{n} x_i\right)^2}{n}}$$

$$a = \bar{y} - b\bar{x}, \quad \text{where } \bar{x} = \frac{\sum_{i=1}^{n} x_i}{n}, \quad \bar{y} = \frac{\sum_{i=1}^{n} y_i}{n}, \tag{7.43}$$

The hypothesis test here is based on the sample regression coefficient b or, more specifically, on $b/\mathrm{SE}(b)$, $\mathrm{SE}(b) \approx S_{yx} / (L_{xx})^{1/2}$. Under the null hypothesis ($H_0 : \beta = 0$), the test statistic $t = \dfrac{b}{\mathrm{SE}(b)}$ follows a t-distribution with $(n-2)$ degrees of freedom. The 95 % CI for β is

$$b \pm t_{0.05/2,\, n-2}\, \mathrm{SE}(b) \tag{7.44}$$

Example 7.7 The annual ASR (World 2010) of lung cancer in men between 1998 and 2007 is listed in Table 7.18. Does the ASR show a change in trend over time?

Table 7.18 ASR of lung cancer between 1998 and 2007

Year	1998	1999	2000	2001	2002	2003	2004	2005	2006	2007
ASR	33.74	35.43	36.77	37.42	33.84	36.51	36.95	36.90	36.80	37.36

The estimated regression line is

$$\hat{Y}(\mathrm{ASR}) = a + bX(\text{year} - 1997)$$

$$n = 10, \quad \sum x_i = 55, \quad \sum x_i^2 = 385, \quad \sum y_i = 361.71, \quad \sum y_i^2 = 13100.57,$$
$$\sum x_i y_i = 2011.48$$

$$b = \frac{\sum x_i y_i - \left(\sum x_i \sum y_i / n\right)}{\sum x_i^2 - \left[\left(\sum x_i\right)^2 / n\right]} = \frac{2011.48 - (55 \times 361.71 / 10)}{385 - (55^2 / 10)} = 0.27$$

$$a = \bar{y} - b\bar{x} = 36.17 - 0.27 \times 5.5 = 34.70$$

(continued)

So, the estimated linear equation is

$$\hat{Y} = 34.70 + 0.27X$$

and

$$SE(b) = \sqrt{\frac{\frac{1}{n-2}\left[\sum(y_i-\bar{y})^2 - b^2\sum(x_i-\bar{x})^2\right]}{\sum(x_i-\bar{x})^2}} = \sqrt{\frac{\frac{1}{10-2}(16.83-0.07\times82.5)}{82.5}} = 0.1288$$

Finally, the 95 % CI for β is:

$$(0.27-1.96\times0.1288,\ 0.27+1.96\times0.1288) = (0.01,\ 0.52)$$

The 95% CI did not include 0, therefore, there is evidence ($\alpha=0.05$) of significant linear association between ASR and time (years), i.e., indicate that each additional year (a one-unit increase) is associated with an increase of 0.27 units of ASR of lung cancer among Beijing men between 1998 and 2007.

Application of the Poisson Regression Model

The main aim of most epidemiological studies is to determine, to the extent possible with the available data, whether an exposure represents a carcinogenic hazard. Because the incidence of cancer is very low and independent in the population, the Poisson log linear regression model is most suitable for describing the relationship between disease incidence and risk factors due to its unique characteristics. Consider the distribution of a number of cancer cases over a long period of time, for example 1 year; assume the probability of a new case occurring on any one day is very small, and the number of cases reported in any two distinct periods of time are independent random variables, then the number of new cases over a 1-year period will follow a Poisson distribution.

Let $Y_1,\ \ldots, Y_n$ be independent random variables with Y_i denoting the number of events observed from exposure n_i for the ith covariate pattern. The Poisson regression model is

$$E(Y_i) = \mu_i = n_i\exp\left(X_i^T\beta\right), \quad Y_i \sim \text{Poisson}(\mu_i) \tag{7.45}$$

The natural link function is the logarithmic function (commonly used in cancer research):

$$\ln \mu_i = \ln n_i + X_i^T\beta \tag{7.46}$$

the term $\ln n_i$ is called the offset. It is a known constant which is readily incorporated into the estimation procedure. As usual, the terms X_i and β describe the covariate pattern and parameters, respectively.

For a binary explanatory variable denoted by an indicator variable, $X_j=0$, if the factor is absent and $X_j=1$ if it is present, the rate ratio (RR) for presence vs. absence is

$$RR = \frac{E\left(Y_i \mid \text{present}, \quad X_j = 1\right)}{E\left(Y_i \mid \text{absent}, \quad X_j = 0\right)} = \exp\left(\beta_j\right) \tag{7.47}$$

provided all the other explanatory variables remain the same. Similarly, for a continuous X_j, a one-unit increase will result in a multiplicative effect of $\exp(\beta_j)$ on the μ. Therefore, parameter estimates are often interpreted on the exponential scale $\exp(\beta)$ in terms of ratio of rates.

The null hypotheses (H_0: $\beta_j=0$) can be tested using the Wald, Score, or likelihood ratio statistics. CIs can be estimated similarly. For example, for parameter β_j :

$$\frac{b_j - \beta_j}{\mathrm{SE}\left(b_j\right)} \sim N\left(0,1\right) \tag{7.48}$$

Residuals are used to check the appropriateness of a chosen response distribution. The residuals for the Poisson distribution are given by $r_i = \left(o_i - e_i\right)/\sqrt{e_i}$, where o_i denotes the observed value of Y_i, and e_i is an estimate of the expected value $E(Y_i)=\mu_i$.

The goodness of fit of a model to data is an important question arising in all statistical modeling. The principles of significance testing, model selection, and diagnostic testing are the same for Poisson regression as for general linear regression; however, the technical details of the methods differ somewhat. There are two common goodness of fit statistic, χ^2 and deviance (D):

$$\chi^2 = \sum r_i = \sum \frac{o_i - e_i}{\sqrt{e_i}}, \quad D = 2\sum\left[o_i \ln\left(o_i / e_i\right) - \left(o_i - e_i\right)\right] \tag{7.49}$$

They are closely related, and both can be used directly as measures of goodness of fit [15].

Example 7.8 Data on smoking and lung cancer deaths are shown in Table 7.19.

Table 7.19 Deaths from lung cancer among urban Chinese men by age and smoking status, 1991

Age class	Smokers			Nonsmokers		
	Deaths	Populations	Death rates/ 10,000	Deaths	Populations	Death rates/ 10,000
35–39	88	1,175,320	0.75	29	681,426	0.43
40–44	118	803,444	1.47	45	554,413	0.81
45–49	260	645,155	4.03	88	455.417	1.95
⋮	⋮	⋮	⋮	⋮	⋮	⋮
65–69	1606	332,614	48.27	355	229,804	15.46
70–74	1364	195,844	69.65	333	155,509	21.43
≥75	1097	154,481	70.99	413	164,176	25.18

(continued)

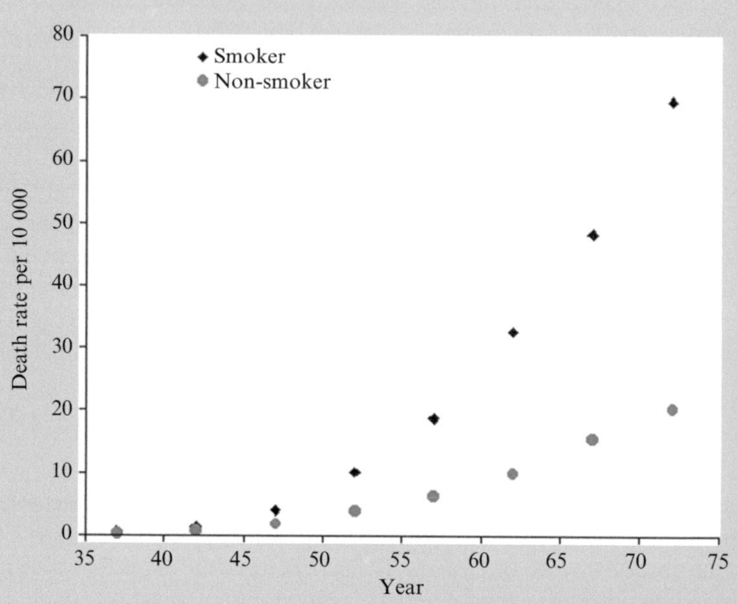

Fig. 7.9 Death rates from lung cancer per 10,000 population for smokers (*diamonds*) and nonsmokers (*dots*)

The data are plotted in Fig. 7.9.

Figure 7.9 shows the clear trend that lung cancer death rates increase with age, but more steeply than in a straight line. Death rates appear to be generally higher among smokers than nonsmokers, but they do not rise as rapidly with age. Various models can be specified to describe these data well. One model, for example, is represented by the form below:

$$\ln\left(\text{deaths}_i\right) = \ln\left(\text{population}_i\right) + \beta_0 + \beta_1 \text{smoke}_i + \beta_2 \text{age}_i \\ + \beta_3 \text{age}_i^2 + \beta_4 \text{smoke}_i \text{age}_i + \beta_5 \text{smoke}_i \text{age}_i^2 \tag{7.50}$$

We may set up different models to examine the age effect only (either a continuous or categorical variable), or to examine the interaction between age and smoking. Some results from this process and the fitted curves for different models are shown in Table 7.20.

Table 7.20 Comparison of Poisson regression models, analysis of deviance

Model	Variance	Deviance	DF	P
A	Intercept	13,779.5332		
B	Smoke	12,211.0727	14	<0.0001
C	Smoke + Age	334.1003	13	<0.0001
D	Smoke + Age + Age^2	44.8679	12	<0.0001
E	Smoke + Age + Age^2 + Smoke × Age^2	19.6306	11	>0.0500
F	Smoke + Age (categorical)	33.4338	7	<0.0001

(continued)

In the analysis of deviance of all selected models, model E revealed adequate fits with 19.63 of deviance on 11 DF for the log link model ($p>0.05$). The final result of the model E is listed below: (Table 7.21)

Table 7.21 Parameter estimates obtained by fitting model E to the data in Table 7.20

Term	Smoke	Age	Age^2	Smoke$\times$Age^2
$\hat{\beta}$	0.50	0.36	−0.0022	0.0001
SE($\hat{\beta}$)	0.1125	0.0136	0.0001	0.0000
Wald statistic	19.95	550.80	277.24	25.48
P-value	<0.0001	<0.0001	<0.0001	<0.0001
Rate ratio	1.65	2.30	0.99	1.00
95 % CI	(0.28, 0.72)	(0.33, 0.39)	(−0.0025, −0.0020)	(0.0001, 0.0002)

Finally, the predictive equation for smoking and lung cancer was:

$$\hat{\mu} = n\exp\left(-21.87 + 0.50X_1(\text{smoke}) + 0.36X_2(\text{age}) - 0.0022X_2^2 + 0.0001X_1X_2^2\right)$$

Since the age effect, X_2, is nonlinear, the effect of a change in age on the lung cancer death rate depends on age. The estimates show that the risk of lung cancer deaths was, on average, about 1.65 times higher for smokers than non-smokers, and smoking will cause more harm for older smokers. Table 7.20 shows that the model fits the data very well.

In this section, we have described the common statistical methods used to analyze cancer registry data, including calculation of statistical indicators in reports, comparison of the incidence in different groups, prediction of time trends, and modeling for etiology analysis. We hope this overview will assist those involved in cancer registries to understand the calculations necessary for the analysis and presentation of their data.

Acknowledgments We are greatly indebted to the data support from Cancer Institute, Chinese Academy of Medical Sciences; School of Public Health, Capital Medical University; and Beijing Office for Cancer Prevention and Control & Beijing Cancer Registry.

We appreciate the useful comments and discussions about parts of this chapter with Professors Hui Li and Susu Liao. We would also like to thank, Yuyan Wang and Zixing Wang, for their assistance during the entire process.

References

1. Hofferkamp J. Standards for completeness, quality, analysis, management, security and confidentiality of data, Standards for cancer registries, vol. 3. Springfield: North American Association of Central Cancer Registries; 2008.

2. Dos Santos SI. Cancer epidemiology: principles and methods. Lyon: World Health Organization; 1999.
3. Fletcher R, Fletcher S. Clinical epidemiology: the essentials. 5th ed. Pennsylvania: Lippincott Williams & Wilkins; 2012.
4. Ahrens W, Pigeot I. Handbook of epidemiology. Berlin: Springer; 2005.
5. Liang W, Lawrence WF, Burnett CB, et al. Acceptability of diagnostic tests for breast cancer. Breast Cancer Res Treat. 2003;79(2):199–206.
6. Siegel R, Ma J, Zou Z, Jemal A. Cancer Statistics, 2014. CA Cancer J Clin. 2014;64(1):9–29.
7. Morabia A, Zhang FF. History of medical screening: from concepts to action. Postgrad Med J. 2014;80(946):463–9.
8. Qiao YL, Sellors JW, Eder PS, et al. A new HPV-DNA test for cervical-cancer screening in developing regions: a cross-sectional study of clinical accuracy in rural China. Lancet Oncol. 2008;9(10):929–36.
9. Kestenbaum B. Epidemiology and biostatistics: an introduction to clinical research. New York: Springer; 2009.
10. Altman DG, Bland JM. Diagnostic tests 3: receiver operating characteristic plots. BMJ. 1994;309(6948):188.
11. Akobeng AK. Understanding diagnostic tests 3: receiver operating characteristic curves. Acta Paediatr. 2007;96(5):644–7.
12. Liu BQ, Peto R, Chen ZM, et al. Emerging tobacco hazards in China: 1. Retrospective proportional mortality study of one million deaths. BMJ. 1998;317(7170):1411–22.
13. Jensen OM, Parkin DM, MacLennan R, et al., editors. Cancer registration: principles and methods. Lyon: International Agency for Research on Cancer; 1991.
14. Armitage P, Berry G. Statistical methods in medical research. 2nd ed. Oxford: Blackwell; 1987.
15. Dobson A, Barnett A. An introduction to generalized linear models. 3rd ed. London: Chapman & Hall; 2008.

Further Reading

Agresti A. An introduction to categorical data analysis. 2nd ed. Hoboken: Wiley; 2007.
Hilsenbeck S, Glaefke G, Feigl P, et al. Quality control for cancer registries. Washington, DC: Department of Health and Human Services; 1985.
Krishnankutty B, Bellary S, Kumar NB, et al. Data management in clinical research: an overview. Indian J Pharmacol. 2012;44(2):168–72.
McFadden E. Management of data in clinical trials. 2nd ed. Inverness: Wiley; 2007.
Newman S. Biostatistical methods in epidemiology. New York: Wiley; 2003.
Prokscha S. Practical guide to clinical data management. 2nd ed. Boca Raton: CRC Press; 2007.
Rondel R, Varley S, Webb C, et al., editors. Clinical data management. 2nd ed. West Sussex: Wiley; 2000.
Rosner B. Fundamentals of biostatistics. 7th ed. Belmont: Thomson-Brooks/Cole; 2006.
Shi Y, Zhang L, Liu X, et al. Icotinib versus gefitinib in previously treated advanced non-small-cell lung cancer (ICOGEN): a randomised, double-blind phase 3 non-inferiority trial. Lancet Oncol. 2013;14:953–61.
Wang D, Bakhai A. Clinical trials—a practical guide to design, analysis, and reporting. London: Remedica; 2006.
Liu X. Survival analysis models and applications. West Sussex: Wiley; 2012.

Chapter 8
Funding for Cancer Research and Clinical Studies in Low- and Middle-Income Countries

John J. Welch and Luis A. Salicrup

Abstract While the majority of new cases of cancers occur in the developing world, cancer research funding is not commensurate with the challenge. The largest funders of cancer research are government institutions in developed countries. While some cancer charities are international in scope, most cancer advocacy and charity organizations also fall within national boundaries. Unlike the situation with infectious diseases, there is no Global Fund to Fight Cancer, and international efforts at coordinating funding are nascent.

Cancer research in developing countries cannot get off the ground without adequate funding to train researchers and equip them to carry out work in both laboratories and in the field.

This chapter addresses resources that can in anyway advance cancer research capacity in these countries: direct funding of investigators or institutions, funding for investigators in well-resourced countries but working on research benefiting developing countries or arrangements where investigators from developed and developing countries work together with joint funding.

Keywords Funding • Professional societies • Charities • Cancer organizations • Grants

Introduction

More than two thirds of cancer deaths worldwide occur in low- and middle-income countries (LMICs) and this proportion will trend upwards in the next decades as their populations expand and age [1]. As most LMICs are struggling to put scarce resources into healthcare delivery, funding for research has taken the back seat, with only a handful of countries committing more than 1 % of GDP to research and development [2]. However, in the absence of evidence-based public health policies based on solid research conducted in local contexts, investments in health delivery

J.J. Welch, M.D., Ph.D. (✉) • L.A. Salicrup, M.S., Ph.D.
Center for Global Health, National Cancer Institute, National Institutes of Health,
9609 Medical Center Drive, Rockville, MD 20850, USA
e-mail: jack.welch@nih.gov

© Springer International Publishing Switzerland 2016
D.C. Stefan (ed.), *Cancer Research and Clinical Trials in Developing Countries*, DOI 10.1007/978-3-319-18443-2_8

will not be effective and the economic burden of non-communicable diseases (NCDs) will threaten long-term prospects for development in these countries [3, 4].

After decades of playing catch up in the field of infectious disease, healthcare systems in LMICs are finally beginning to pull even with the challenges of HIV/ AIDS, malaria, tuberculosis, and other tropical and childhood infectious diseases. Massive national and international investments in research have yielded effective public health interventions that will spare future generations from these diseases. Based on that experience, the world health community is poised for the first time to get ahead of the curve by injecting funding into NCD research before these diseases peak. Infectious diseases will still be a concern in LMICs for decades to come and funding for research in those areas will be needed, but even now, there is recognition that the research infrastructure and funding relationships put in place to address infectious diseases should start to be leveraged to serve broader health issues.

While the majority of new cases of cancers occur in the developing world and will do even more so in the future, it is safe to say that cancer research funding is not commensurate with the challenge. The largest funders of cancer research are government institutions in developed countries. Although these institutions may have foreign components, their funding base is national in nature and they must answer to that constituency, concentrating on domestic programs. While some cancer charities are international in scope, most cancer advocacy and charity organizations also fall within national boundaries. Unlike the situation with infectious diseases, there is no Global Fund to Fight Cancer, and international efforts at coordinating funding are nascent.

Intent of This Chapter

Cancer research in LMICs cannot get off the ground without adequate funding to train researchers and equip them to carry out work in both laboratories and in the field. This chapter addresses resources that can in anyway advance cancer research capacity in LMICs: direct funding of investigators or institutions in LMICs; funding for investigators in well-resourced countries but working on research benefiting LMICs; or arrangements where investigators from LMIC and well-resourced countries work together with joint funding.

This chapter follows the World Bank classification of economies; in the most recent classification of 214 economies evaluated, 34 were classified as low, 50 as lower-middle, 55 as upper-middle, and the remainder as high income [5]. This scheme is not ideal as it does not capture wealth inequities within countries that may translate to areas of high and low healthcare needs within one country, but it is a widely used system and a useful starting point [6].

Within the middle-income bracket, this chapter emphasizes external funding aimed at the lower-middle bracket, as some of the upper-middle income countries have established their own funding mechanisms and are themselves reaching out as donor countries. There is also a bias in this chapter towards the younger investigator, who may need particular attention in terms of training or in obtaining a first grant that could pave the way to a productive career. It is assumed that more senior investigators will already have a better grasp of the funding landscape and, presumably, also have a stake in finding funding for their junior colleagues. Similarly, this chapter will emphasize general funding sources rather than those narrowly focused by disease or geographic area; again, it is presumed that researchers will be familiar with funding opportunities within their own countries and subspecialties.

In addition to training, the chapter focuses on funding for research to guide cancer control planning and applied efforts in a region; research to identify gaps in cancer care delivery within public health systems; clinical trials; and implementation science. While translational research is considered, the chapter will not examine funding for basic laboratory research, early phase clinical research (except for pilots), or funding for general health system improvement or training of allied health professionals.

Grant Writing Advice

The goal in academic research is to maintain a portfolio of grants with sufficient overlap to maintain continuity of funding. Over a career of writing such grants, senior investigators acquire useful grantsmanship skills, and junior investigators are advised to seek their assistance in preparing grants. The art of preparing funding proposals is beyond the scope of this chapter, but beginning investigators may wish to review advice from the South African Medical Research Council (SAMRC) (South African MRC) and in the Grants Processes chapter of the WHO and AORTIC's Handbook for Cancer Research in Africa [6].

Even seasoned grant writers may need occasional reminders about good grant practices, so the following tips are offered (Table 8.1):

Proposals submitted by or on behalf of investigators in LMICs should anticipate some funder concerns including administrative accountability and financial transparency. To maximize their return on investment in research, donors will favor openness about and publication of all study results, even the negative ones. Finally, remember that donors do not want to be donors forever; proposals should address the long-term sustainability of proposed research.

Funding Portals

A key to finding funding is figuring out which funding sources are already operating in an area and what sort of research they are funding. Three web-based portals aggregate research funding information across multiple donors.

Table 8.1 Tips for good grant writing practices

Do	Don't
… Closely read the call for funding. Is your project a reasonable fit? Is your proposal responsive to the call?	… Submit proposals that are not on topic or that duplicate already funded work
… Make sure the call is current	… Send your proposal in past the deadline
… Assure that all the regulatory boxes are ticked—compliance with national laws, ethics review, human subjects projection, animal welfare, intellectual property requirements, publication agreements, and so on	… Make the reviewer's job a chore—write clearly, proofread (if necessary, enlist a native speaker), write concisely, don't make the reviewer search for figures or references; be careful not to carry over irrelevant material when pasting
… Include required materials and comply with all instructions in the call for funding	… Gloss over the science—provide preliminary data, support assertions; be quantitative, provide methodological and statistical plans
… Clearly delineate the aims of the project, the deliverables, and the timeframe	… Rush on preparation of the budget. The budget may not be an interesting part of the grant, but reviewers will scrutinize it
… Talk to someone who has successfully obtained funding from the same or a similar source	… Fail to give the big picture; how does this research benefit public health and advance development?

World RePORT

The World RePORT database (http://worldreport.nih.gov/) is an attempt to improve coordination of international funding by pooling biomedical research funding data from multiple donors. The database contains information submitted by the HIROs (Heads of International Research Organizations) group: the Bill and Melinda Gates Foundation, the Canadian Institutes of Health Research (CIHR), the European Commission's Directorate General for Research and Innovation, the European and Developing Countries Clinical Trials Partnership (EDCTP), the French National Institute for Health and Medical Research (INSERM), the Max-Planck-Gesellschaft, the UK Medical Research Council (MRC), the US National Institutes of Health, the Institut Pasteur, the Swedish International Development and Cooperation Agency (SIDA), and the Wellcome Trust [7].

Presently, only programs in Sub-Saharan Africa have been added to the database and the website is marked "beta" to indicate that additional funding agencies, wider geographic coverage, and additional programmatic features are expected in the future. One aspect that is notably lacking from the site is award amounts; it is possible to determine how many projects have been awarded to a given country, but the dollar amount is not recorded in the dataset, although external links are provided that in some cases point towards this information. When a single grant is awarded to multiple sites in a recipient country, these are counted as separate projects in the database.

Some observations from the 2013 dataset may be useful to researchers seeking funding in LMICs because the dataset provides some insight into the donors and

Table 8.2 WorldRePORT 2013 dataset

Country	Population	Projects	Projects per 1,000,000 population	Economy
South Africa	48,375,645	539	11.14	Upper-middle
Uganda	35,918,915	389	10.83	Low
Kenya	45,010,056	339	7.53	Low
United Republic of Tanzania	49,639,138	199	4.01	Low
Malawi	17,377,468	121	6.96	Low
Nigeria	177,155,754	112	0.63	Lower-middle
Ghana	25,758,108	90	3.49	Lower-middle
Zambia	14,638,505	89	6.08	Lower-middle
Ethiopia	96,633,458	74	0.77	Low
Zimbabwe	13,771,721	66	4.79	Low
Gambia, The	1,925,527	63	32.72	Low
Cameroon	23,130,708	55	2.38	Lower-middle
Burkina Faso	18,365,123	53	2.89	Low
Mali	16,455,903	52	3.16	Low
Mozambique	24,692,144	46	1.86	Low
Botswana	2,155,784	45	20.87	Upper-middle
Côte d'Ivoire	22,848,945	34	1.49	Lower-middle
Senegal	13,635,927	34	2.49	Lower-middle
DR Congo	77,433,744	32	0.41	Low

their priorities. The first observation is that researchers in countries where English is an official language have a strong advantage in obtaining funding; this likely reflects the higher proportion of funding from English-speaking donor organizations and the use of English as a common medium for applying for funding. To maximize funding opportunities, cancer researchers who are not comfortable working in English should find colleagues skilled in the language to help them track down opportunities and prepare submissions (Table 8.2).

Of the top twelve countries by number of projects, only Ethiopia does not have English as an official language. Francophone countries fall in the low to mid-range, with one project in Burundi and Togo and up to 55 in Cameroon. Aside from 46 projects in Mozambique, lusopohone countries have few projects: Guinea-Bissau has five, but Angola, Cape Verde, and São Tomé have none. Arabic-language countries are mostly in Northern Africa and their data are not captured in the HIROs dataset; however, of the Arabic-speaking countries in Sub-Saharan Africa, Chad and Eritrea have one project, and Comoros, Djibouti, and Mauritania have none.

South Africa, an upper-middle-income country, heads the list. Its top ranking may reflect the preference of some donors to work with more established infrastructure; the prevalence of HIV/AIDS-related funding is also a major factor. Despite the predominance of projects in South Africa, most projects were awarded to countries at the lower end of the economic spectrum (Table 8.3).

Table 8.3 Projects per economy type in Sub-Saharan Africa (excluding South Africa)

Economy	Population	Projects	Projects per million
High	722,254	0	0.00
Upper-middle	26,537,698	94	3.54
Lower-middle	290,247,972	430	1.48
Low	535,405,887	1544	2.88

Table 8.4 Projects per subject

[a]Country	Cancer	Non-HIV cancers	HIV, AIDS	TB	Malaria	Neglected tropic diseases	Maternal, child, reproductive
Uganda	18	9	219	78	37	10	56
Kenya	17	12	118	3	55	14	84
South Africa	16	9	239	90	10	0	96
Zambia	9	2	37	4	7	0	22
Nigeria	7	3	37	5	8	1	7
Ghana	7	6	12	4	10	5	12
Tanzania	6	5	58	20	32	3	45
Malawi	6	4	46	7	25	1	24
Gambia, The	5	5	8	11	18	0	14
Zimbabwe	3	0	36	14	1	0	9
Rwanda	3	0	15	2	1	0	7
Senegal	2	2	11	5	9	2	3
Botswana	1	1	36	2	0	0	11
Cameroon	1	0	24	9	11	4	2
Ethiopia	1	1	20	12	0	2	6
Burkino Faso	1	0	17	4	21	2	17
Congo (DRC)	1	1	16	2	2	0	3

[a]Countries with no cancer-related projects are not included on this list. Some projects fall into multiple categories

A breakdown of project type into categories based on project titles puts the amount of funding dedicated to cancer research into perspective and also underlines the extent to which cancer studies in Africa are tied to HIV/AIDS research (Table 8.4):

Looking only at cancer-specific projects, it is clear that of the HIROs institutions, the US National Institutes of Health and its collaborators fund the bulk of projects in Sub-Saharan Africa (Table 8.5):

The International Cancer Research Partnership

The International Cancer Research Partnership (ICRP) was established in 2000 to assist in the strategic coordination of global funding and collaboration for cancer research. Member organizations submit funding data classified according to the

Table 8.5 Cancer-related projects in SSA by donor

Summary: HIROs 2013 cancer-related projects in SSA by donor		
EC	5	2 in South Africa; 1 in Burkino Faso, Gambia, Nigeria
INSERM	4	2 Gambia, 1 Congo (DRC), 1 Nigeria
MRC	1	1 Gambia
NIH/NIH Collaboration	88	17 Kenya; 14 South Africa, Uganda; 9 Zambia; 7 Ghana; 6 Malawi; 5 Nigeria, Tanzania; 3 Rwanda, Zimbabwe, 2 Senegal, 1 Gambia; 1 Botswana; 1 Cameroon; 1 Ethiopia
SIDA	1	Uganda
Wellcome	1	Tanzania
Total	100	

Common Scientific Outline (CSO) to facilitate database searching. Currently, the database contains data on more than 60,000 grants from 81 organizations from Australia, Canada, France, Japan, the Netherlands, the UK, and the USA. Data can be sorted according to the CSO, text words, funding or recipient organization, or recipient geography. Projects can be classified according to type of cancer or project (clinical trials, research or training) [8].

The dataset from fiscal year 2013 contains 12,096 projects; however, 12,089 of these are in high-income economies. The remaining projects include one in a low-income country, Malawi, one in a low-middle income country, India, and one each in upper-middle income countries: Argentina, China, Costa Rica, Thailand, and South Africa. While the ICRP dataset is cancer-specific and global, the HIROs dataset in the World RePORT is more comprehensive, but does not flag whether projects are cancer-specific. Like the HIROs dataset, the ICRP dataset does not include funding levels, but does provide links to award documents.

Looking at a decade's worth of funding data (2004–2014), the ICRP database identified 57,036 awards: 31 in low- and low-middle-income countries. Since funders appear in this dataset that are not captured by HIROs, investigators should check both. In addition to identifying donors, investigators may find it helpful to consult the databases to find in-country or international collaborators who have received past awards (Table 8.6).

Global Oncology Cancer Resource Map

Global Oncology, Inc., a US-based not-for-profit organization has announced the creation of a web-based tool to map international cancer research, cancer care, and cancer outreach programs globally to facilitate collaboration and align international efforts. The site launched in 2015 [9].

Table 8.6 Countries funded per donor

Income	Countries	Funders
Low	Malawi	US NCI (1)
	The Gambia	UK MRC (14)[a]
Low-middle	Egypt	Avon (1), US NCI (1)
	Guatemala	AICR (1)
	India	AICR (1), US DOD (1), Komen, NCI (4), Wellcome (4)
	Senegal	US NCI (1)
Upper-middle	Argentina	Komen (3), US NCI (3)
	American Samoa	US NCI (3)
	Brazil	US NCI (2), Wellcome (2)
	China	AICR (1), US NCI (7), ONSF (1)
	Costa Rica	US NCI (2)
	Hungary	Wellcome (4)
	Mexico	AICR (1), Avon (3), US NCI (1)
	Thailand	ONSF (1), Wellcome (1)
	South Africa	US NCI (3), Wellcome (2)

AICR American Institute for Cancer Research, *Avon* Avon Foundation for Women, *Komen* The Susan G. Komen Foundation, *ONSF* Oncology Nursing Society Foundation; *US NCI* US National Cancer Institute, *US DOD* US Department of Defense, *Wellcome* Wellcome Trust
[a]Some of these represent the same project funded in multiple years

Governments

Governments and government-associated institutions are the largest contributors to global health research funding, for cancer even more so than for infectious diseases, where international organizations and charities play a stronger role. The emerging BRICS economies, Brazil, Russia, India, China, and South Africa, have greatly expanded their roles in global health assistance in the last decade [10] and are similarly stepping up their commitment to biomedical research funding, often through South–South collaborations [11].

Brazil

National Council for Scientific and Technological Development

The Conselho Nacional de Desenvolvimento Científico e Tecnológico (CNPq) within the Brazilian Ministry of Science, Technology, and Innovation promotes scientific and technological research and training of researchers. The Council offers research scholarships for Brazilian students studying both in country and abroad from high school through postgraduate levels of education. These opportunities are detailed on the CNPq website [12].

The Brazil Scientific Mobility Program (BSMP), formally known as Science without Borders, sponsored by CAPES (Coordenação de Aperfeiçoamento de Pessoal de Nível Superior) and CNPq, supports fellowships for Brazilian students to study in the United States. In addition to these programs, CNPq works alongside the World Academy of Sciences (TWAS) to support a postgraduate fellowship program, which allows young scientists from developing countries other than Brazil to pursue doctoral research in the natural sciences at Brazilian universities [13].

Canada

International Development Research Centre

The International Development Research Centre (IDRC) is a Canadian Federal Crown Corporation established in 1970 by an Act of Parliament. Although based in Ottawa, Canada, the IDRC has regional offices in Kenya, Egypt, India, and Uruguay. The IDRC receives most of its annual appropriation from the Canadian Parliament, but international government and private charitable donors also contribute. The mission is to find long-term solutions to problems in the developing world through research.

Masters or doctoral level students from LMICs may apply for International Fellowships in fields that support IDRC thematic priorities, which include Agriculture and Environment, Global Health Policy, Science and Innovation, and Social and Economic Policy. In contrast to many government-supported educational grants, these fellowships do not require the applicant to study at an institution in the awarding country, but rather at a partner university in a developing country. Note that this is an externally directed award; Canadian citizens are not eligible. A listing of currently available awards and partner institutions is available on the IDRC website [14].

The IDRC also offers 1 year of support for researchers in the process of completing or having completed masters or doctoral-level training at a recognized university. Canadian citizens and permanent residents are eligible for this award in addition to citizens of developing countries. The awards focus on research conducted in one or more developing countries; research in some countries is not supported, while in other countries prior approval must be sought [15].

Canadian Institutes of Health Research

The CIHR was created in 2000 by an Act of Parliament and is Canada's health research investment agency. The CIHR provides funding to Canadian citizens and residents with award programs for students at masters and doctoral level as well as postdoctoral research fellowship and incentive awards for physician-scientists.

In general, these awards are not thematic in nature, but meant to broadly support the development of academic researchers in Canada. While the awardee must be Canadian, the research may be directed towards LMICs. Additionally, the doctoral award provides supplemental funding for research conducted outside of Canada [16].

Global Health Research Initiative

The IDRC, the Department of Foreign Affairs, Trade, and Development, and the CIHR have partnered to create the Global Health Research Initiative (GHRI) to address pressing problems in the developing world. The calls for proposal tend to be relatively broad in nature, so cancer research may be a suitable component in a project submission [17].

China

Ministry of Science and Technology

The National Health and Family Planning Commission of the People's Republic of China (formerly, the Ministry of Health) is primarily focused on healthcare provision and internal medical policy and programs, but the Ministry of Science and Technology (MoST) has substantial involvement in international scientific exchange and cooperation, including promotion of South–South partnerships. These partnerships are administered through its Department of International Cooperation [18]. The Department has initiated two science and technology partnership programs, one with ASEAN [19] and one directed towards Africa [20]. Both programs tie into the MoST's Talented Young Scientist Program, which supports the work of young scientists at Chinese research institutes, universities, and enterprises [21].

National Natural Science Foundation of China

The National Natural Science Foundation of China (NSFC) was founded in 1986 under jurisdiction of the Chinese State Council and administers the Natural Science Fund on behalf of the central government. Its operating budget in 2012 was 80 CN¥ million. The foundation encourages international cooperation and scientific exchange and has partnered with 35 countries and regions [22] including a number of LMICs such as Belarus, Bulgaria, Egypt, India, Mexico, Pakistan, the Philippines, and Thailand; scientists in these countries may contact NSFC regarding exchange opportunities via their respective national organizations that have partnered with NSFC [23]. The NSFC maintains a research fund for international young postdoctoral scientists to support 6–12-month study at Chinese institutions; application is made via Chinese host institutions [24].

Chinese Academy of Sciences

The Chinese Academy of Sciences (CAS) was established in 1949 and is the home of most Big Science in China. Part of its mission includes international collaboration and graduate training in science and technology. Under the CAS President's International Fellowship Initiative (PIFI), the academy administers several fellowship programs, which bring young and senior international scientists to study in China. Since 2004, CAS has also offered the CAS-TWAS Fellowship, which supports 200 international graduate students from LMICs to undertake research at CAS institutes each year [25].

Chinese Scholarship Council

The Chinese Scholarship Council (CSC) is a non-profit institution affiliated to the Ministry of Education. With different types of funding programs, it offers financial support to Chinese citizens studying abroad and to international students and scholars studying in China. A number of Chinese-government-sponsored scholarships are offered through CSC including a series of bilateral programs with specific partner governments; a general program for graduate students who wish to study at designated Chinese universities; and, two regional programs, one directed at graduate students in the ASEAN University Network and another for students from Pacific Island countries. CSC also administers the UNESCO Great Wall Fellowship program, through which the government of China supports study by 25 graduate students and senior scholars at Chinese institutions [26]. These 1-year fellowships are directed to developing UNESCO member states in Africa, Asia-Pacific, and some Arab States [27].

European Union

The EC DG for Research and Innovation oversees funding for scientific research within the European Union (EU). Multi-year funding plans have in the past been called framework programs, although the current one is designated Horizon 2020. Horizon 2020 has been funded at the level of 80€ billion and covers the period from

2014 to 2020. For those not easily frightened by complexity, an online manual is available to help researchers navigate the many funding opportunities within this program [28]. Calls for funding across all Horizon 2020 programs are consolidated at a single website [28]. The three programs most relevant to cancer research in LMICs are highlighted below.

Marie Skłodowska-Curie Actions

Programs supporting early career development and training are collected in this program, which comes under the "Excellent Science" pillar of Horizon 2020. The Marie Skłodowska-Curie Actions (MSCA) supports the mobility of researchers moving to Europe for training (European Fellowships) and conversely provides funding for European investigators to spend time visiting research institutions outside Europe. In both cases, these fellowships are directed at individuals with at least 4 years postdoctoral experience [29]. The postdoctoral fellowships offered by the IARC (see below) are in part supported by this and other EU sources.

European Research Council

The European Research Council (ERC) was created by the European Commission in 2007 under the seventh framework program to support European basic research across a broad range of subject areas. The total budget allocation for 2014–2020 under Horizon 2020 is 13.1€ billion. The ERC offers a series of competitive grants targeted to investigators at various stages of career development, plus other programs to support pilot projects or provide gap funding to bring mature research to market. The success rate for grant applicants in 2013 ranged from 3 % for synergy grants to 24 % for proof of concept grants; starting and advanced career grants were funded at 9.2 % and 12.3 %, respectively [30].

Funding mechanisms are described on the ERC website [31]. Funding proposals must be submitted in response to open calls [32]. European-based researchers can apply, but researchers from outside Europe are also eligible for funding, if their research is based at a host institution in an EU member state or associated country for the award period.

European and Developing Countries Clinical Trial Partnership

The European and Developing Countries Clinical Trial Partnership (EDCTP) was initially launched in 2003 as a 600€ million, 5-year program to enable conduct of clinical trials addressing AIDS, malaria, and tuberculosis in developing countries. The partnership leverages resources from the EU, Norway, Switzerland, pharmaceutical, and charity donors. In December 2014, the 1.4€ billion second phase of the partnership was announced. The program will continue to support early and late phase clinical trial development on the three primary diseases, plus neglected infectious diseases, and to promote multicenter clinical trial collaborations and capacity development in sub-Saharan Africa. While cancer research is not specifically supported, infrastructural support, strengthening of ethical and regulatory frameworks, training and career development, and better intra-Africa collaboration should have collateral benefits for cancer research. In the initial program, more projects were non-disease-specific than were dedicated to the targeted diseases. More germane to cancer research in LMICs, the partnership could address clinical prevention or research trials for cancers etiologically due to or associated with endemic infections such as HIV, human papilloma virus, Epstein Barr virus, hepatitis viruses, and enteric infections that promote cancer-associated inflammation.

Funding calls are announced online [33] and have included fellowship funding for individuals as well as institutional and network grants.

France

Institut National de la Santé et de la Recherche Médicale

Institut National de la Santé et de la Recherche Médicale (INSERM) falls administratively under the French Ministry of Health and Social Affairs and the Ministry of Research. The institute's 2014 budget was 866.6€ million, 70 % from the state, and 30 % from external sources. Cancer research is a core theme; 16 % of the budget and 37 research units are dedicated to cancer research. According to 2013 World RePORT data, INSERM supported four projects in Sub-Saharan Africa through institutional collaborations. Current calls for scientific projects and cooperation can be found online [34]. In addition, INSERM maintains a number of bilateral cooperative agreements [35] with several countries that provide for reciprocal short-term visits, seminars, and postdoctoral placements. Finally, INSERM provides some practical advice for investigators interested in performing research at INSERM [36] and for obtaining support for travel and other expenses for researchers from specific countries [37] (Fig. 8.1).

Institut National du Cancer de France

Institut National du Cancer de France (INCa-Fr) was created in 2004 as the government agency in charge of coordinating the fight against cancer, including development of a scientific program, review, and financing of research proposals. The yearly budget of INCa-Fr is about 105€ million (2013 figures) [39]. Administratively, INCa-Fr falls under the Ministry of Health and Social Affairs and the Ministry of

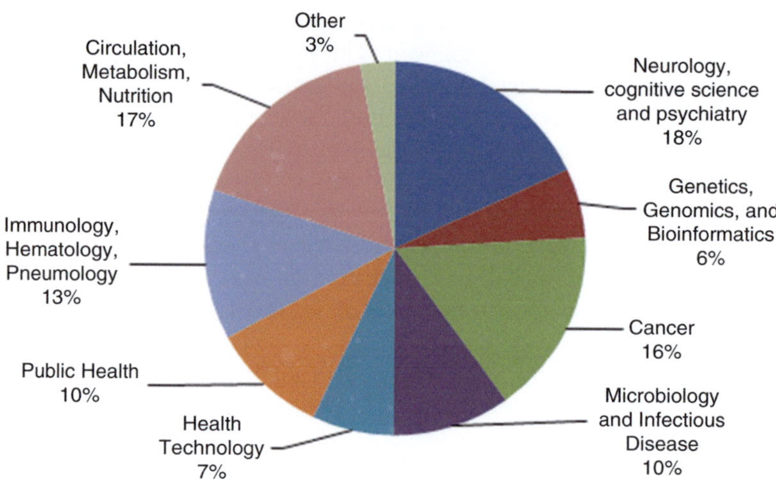

Fig. 8.1 INSERM expenditures in 2014 by research area. Adapted from the 2014 INSERM budget [38]

Higher Education and Research. The institute is responsible for implementing the Plan Cancer, a 5-year road map of cancer priorities for France. Although global health and international development are not singled out as objectives under this plan, several plan priorities such as tobacco control and cancer prevention and screening are global in nature. INCa-Fr is involved in cancer research in the developing world through partnerships with organizations such as the WHO's International Agency for Research on Cancer, the International Atomic Energy Agency, the UICC, the International Cancer Cooperation Network, and the INCTR (the International Network for Cancer Treatment and its French branch, the AMCC, L'Alliance Mondiale Contre le Cancer). In terms of capacity building and training, INCa-Fr has worked on a ministry-to-ministry basis to establish collaborations with institutions in Senegal and Mauritania. The INCa-Fr website also provides links to French partner sites, which fund cancer research [40].

In terms of direct calls for funding, INCa-Fr oversees the selection of projects financed both by the institute itself and by French regional health agencies (ARS, les Agences Régionales de Santé). Applications for both institution and project-specific funding are available online [41] (Fig. 8.2).

India

Indian Council of Medical Research

The Indian Council of Medical Research (IMRC) falls under the Indian Ministry of Health and Family Welfare's Department of Health Research and supports biomedical research through intra- and extramural programs. Intramural research is conducted at

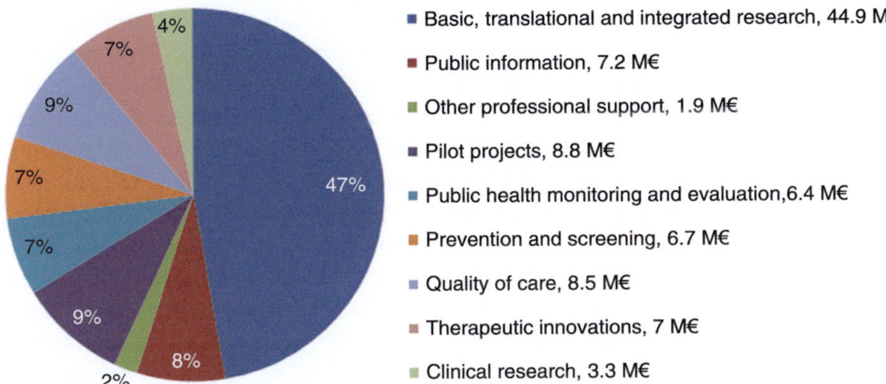

Fig. 8.2 INCa-Fr budgetary outlays for 2013 by subject area. Adapted from the 2013 INCa-Fr budget [39]

the Council's 32 national research institutes, centers, and units. Extramural research is implemented through academic centers and institutions. The Council has designated NCDs including cancer as a thrust area [42].

The Council has established a number of bilateral memoranda of understanding with research institutions worldwide, which may avail Indian researchers of opportunities for scientific exchange and collaboration [43]. The Council supports a number of student and professional research fellowships. Their International Fellowship Program for Indian Biomedical Scientists supports young or senior scientists at the M.D. or Ph.D. level to perform research work abroad [44], while their International Fellowship Program for Biomedical Scientists from Developing Countries supports 1- to 6-month fellowships for researchers with at least a Master of Science or M.B.B.S. degree; application for these fellowships should be submitted through the Indian mission in the researcher's home country [45].

South Africa

South African Medical Research Council

The SAMRC was established in 1969 with the remit of promoting improvement in health and quality of life in South Africa. While its programs are primarily national in scope (the 1991 South African Medical Research Council Act [46] does provide for research outside of South Africa), investigators in the sub-Saharan region are likely to find oncological issues that are regional in nature, but may be addressed by SAMRC resources. The SAMRC has both intra- and extramural programs. Although none of the intramural units are specific to oncology, several address research areas relevant to cancer: tobacco, statistical methodology, environmental exposures, and NCDs. Within the extramural program, there is a unit explicitly dedicated to cancer epidemiology and a number of others that address basic and clinical aspects of oncology. South African citizens pursuing masters or doctoral level training in the health sciences may review available training and career development opportunities on the SAMRC website [47]. For self-initiated research grants, current guidelines require that applicants have completed the equivalent of a Ph.D., are employed at a recognized research institution, and are either a South African citizen or permanent resident. Full guidelines and application materials for these self-initiated grants are provided online [48]. According to the 2014 Annual Performance Plan, the FY 2012/13 budget totaled 577 million Rand, with 406 million devoted to core research [49].

Finally, SAMRC maintains a useful listing of funding opportunities available from external sources. While aimed at SAMRC investigators, this list is well-maintained and provides up-to-date pointers to additional funding sources, many of which are useful for cancer researchers [50]. The South African government recognizes that some of its commitments to collaborating organizations within the Southern African Development Community, African Union, and WHO are likely to be affected through the SAMRC [51], so it seems likely that cross-border funding options will improve in the future. To that end, the Council provides grants to host national or international conferences [52].

Russia

Российский Научный Фонд

The Russian Science Fund offers competitive institutional grants for subject areas ranging from maths and computer science through life science, space research, engineering, and social science [53]. These awards are primarily aimed at researchers in the Russian Federation, but according to the results from the most recent call for international scientific project support [54], applications included about equal numbers of Russian and international investigators for projects in 23 countries. Most of the collaborations were with researchers in Germany, UK, and US, although the list includes some middle-income countries such as China, Mexico, and Ukraine.

Российский Фонд Фундаментальных Исследований

The Russian Fund for Fundamental Research, founded in 1992, is a non-profit federal institution of the Russian Federation. As its name suggests, the fund supports basic research including biological and medical research. The fund also promotes international cooperation through agreements with organizations in twenty five countries, with some emphasis on relations with Member States in the Commonwealth of Independent States (CIS) [55]. Of the about 8 billion Ruble 2013 budget, 355 million was allocated to international projects, and 100 million to projects in CIS countries [56].

A new funding opportunity was launched in 2013, a fellowship for young foreign scientists to conduct research at scientific institutions in the Russian Federation; 178 applications from 35 countries were received for this opportunity, 130 of the applicants were from CIS member states, the remainder for more distant countries including a number of LMICs that are not CIS members: Argentina, Bulgaria, China, Cuba, Georgia, India, Mongolia, Serbia, and Ukraine. In total, 111 projects were supported. Additionally, there were 22 calls for international scientific collaborations in the same year, with 310 projects supported including bilateral projects involving LMIC investigators in Armenia, Belorussia, Kyrgyzstan, India, China, Mongolia, and Ukraine [57].

The Fund offers a number of calls for funding, many of which are bilateral funding announcements for joint projects with counterpart institutions, for example, TUBITAK in Turkey, or the Department of Science and Technology in India [58].

Sweden

Swedish International Development Corporation

Swedish International Development Corporation (SIDA) works in a limited number of countries in Eastern Europe, Africa, and Asia according to the Swedish government's strategy for developmental assistance. Presently, SIDA commits SEK 2 billion per year to healthcare access in poor countries. While SIDA traditionally focused on infectious diseases, it recognizes that NCDs constitute a growing concern. SIDA does not fund individuals to start private projects; rather, it partners with NGOs and public and private sector institutions. Because SIDA cannot directly fund non-Swedish CSOs, external CSOs may consider partnering with a Swedish counterpart. Research institutions in a limited number of countries (Bolivia, Burkina Faso, Ethiopia, Mozambique, Rwanda, Tanzania, and Uganda) may apply for direct funding via the Secretariat for Research Cooperation. Specific programs are aimed at creating research and training linkages between institutions in these countries and their Swedish counterparts. The research cooperation web portal [59] lists open calls and provides helpful information about the application process. A number of projects administered by TWAS, below, are funded in partnership with SIDA.

Turkey

The Scientific and Technological Research Council of Turkey

Scientific and Technological Research Council of Turkey (TUBITAK) was established in 1963 to promote, develop, and coordinate overall research and development funding in the fields of social and natural sciences. TUBITAK's current budget is approximately $2.5 million, of which 11 % supports health and biomedical research and 36 % supports natural sciences research projects including molecular biology, immunology, genetics, bioengineering, and other disciplines. The average annual award per project from TUBITAK is 360,000 Turkish Lira (about $180,000).

According to the Vision 2013 road map for Turkey's transition from a middle- to high-income economy, TUBITAK is responsible for development in areas of science and technology. To promote capacity building, the council supports national and international scholarships and fellowships, and research support for scientists early in their careers [60].

United Kingdom

UK Medical Research Council

Global Health is one of the six science strategy areas for the UK MRC, a government agency that guides the country's medical strategy. The UK MRC's global health portfolio currently receives about £48 million per year in funding. While the portfolio is heavily weighted towards infectious diseases, particularly HIV/AIDS [61], UK MRC is placing increasing emphasis on NCDs; even so, only one out of 187 projects in the most recent portfolio report was directed at cancer research [62]. Most of the focus in global health has been directed towards Africa, which is not surprising given that there are permanent MRC research units in The Gambia and Uganda.

In addition to project-specific funding, the UK MRC sponsors fellowships and studentships. These awards are limited to UK residents, although there are provisions that allow some fellowship research to be conducted abroad. The MRC has established strategic partnerships that extend their ability to support research in the NCD arena. These include an agreement with the UK Department for Development (DFID), which has dedicated £90 million for the 5-year period (2013–2018) to fund areas of mutual interest including capacity development, translational and implementation research, public health research, health services research, and include provisions to fund large-scale trials. The MRC/DFID concordat has funded African Research Leaders programs in Ghana, South Africa, Burkina Faso, Uganda, Kenya, and Nigeria. Other MRC partnerships include the European and Developing

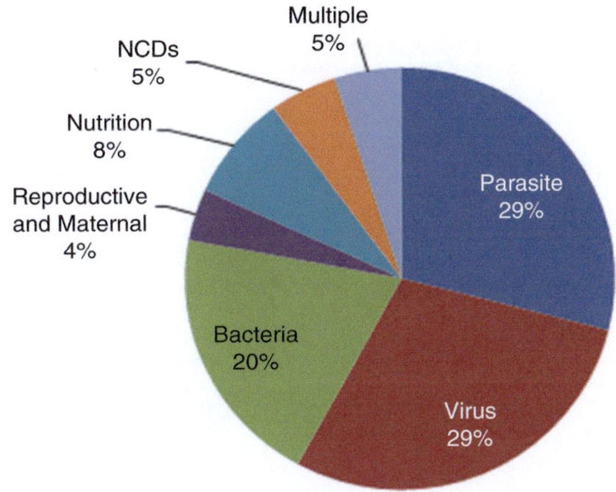

Fig. 8.3 UK MRC budget allocation in 2012–13 by research area [64]

Countries Clinical Trials Partnership (EDCTP, see above), which has supported vaccine trials in Africa, and the Global Alliance for Chronic Diseases, a multination partnership aimed at supporting research in NCDs [63] (Fig. 8.3).

United States of America

In 2009, American President Barack Obama launched the $63 billion Global Health Initiative [65], which underlined the government's commitment to global health and built on the success of previous initiatives such as the President's Emergency Plan for AIDS Relief (PEPFAR) [66]. Health research is funded primarily through the National Institutes of Health (NIH), while development-related research is supported by the United States Agency for International Development, USAID.

The National Institutes of Health

The NIH was established in 1887 and falls administratively under the US Department of Health and Human Services. The NIH is made up of 27 institutes and centers, two of which are particularly relevant for global cancer research: the US National Cancer Institute (NCI) and the Fogarty International Center, both discussed in more detail below. Each year, the NIH invests about $30.1 billion in medical research. Eighty per cent of that funding is awarded through almost 50,000 competitive grants to more than 300,000 researchers at more than 2,500 universities, medical schools, and research institutions nationally and around the world. Current and past funding by NIH can be examined through an online tool [67], which allows sorting of funding data by location (Fig. 8.4).

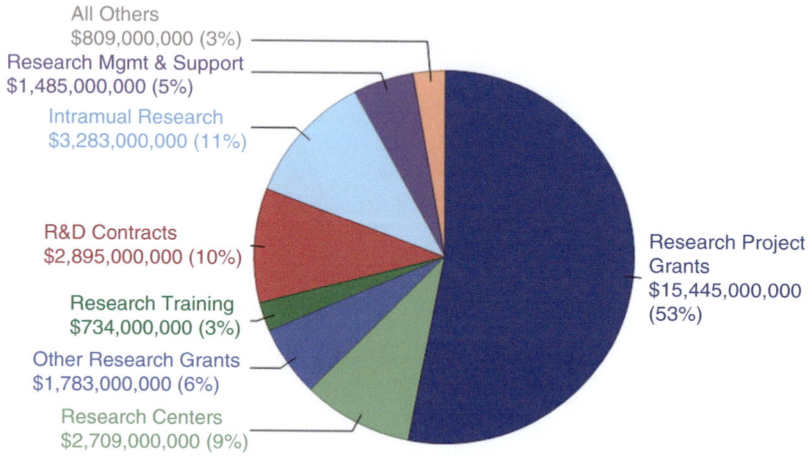

Fig. 8.4 The 2015 budget request from NIH. More than half the budget is dedicated to research project grants (RPGs) to individuals and institutions, most of which are domestic, but some foreign. Most funding for investigators from LMICs comes through collaboration with recipients of RPGs located at NCI-supported academic institutions or on the NIH campus [68]

US National Cancer Institute

The NCI was established within the NIH by the National Cancer Institute Act of 1937 [69]. Its mission is to eliminate suffering and death due to cancer. With a budget of around $5 billion per year, the NCI is the best funded of the NIH institutes. In 2012, about 42 % of funds were allocated for 5,021 Research Project Grants. These grants are extremely competitive; only about seven per cent of proposals for the most common research projects grants, R01 grants, were funded.

About 17 % of research at NCI is conducted through the intramural program. Although this section of NCI does not award grants, a substantial number of projects, in epidemiology for example, involve collaboration with cancer researchers in LMICs, so it is still worthwhile reviewing intramural research efforts. All grant funding, however, stems from the NCI extramural programs, which can award grants to US or international investigators.

The extramural grant portal [70] provides an overview of the basics of the grant application process and the types of grants available as well as application forms. This site includes step-by-step guidance through grant preparation and submission, but also lays out the timeline of what to expect during the review process, at the time of award, and how to administer the grant during its lifetime and at its end. Information specific to foreign grant applicants is also provided [71] (Figs. 8.5 and 8.6).

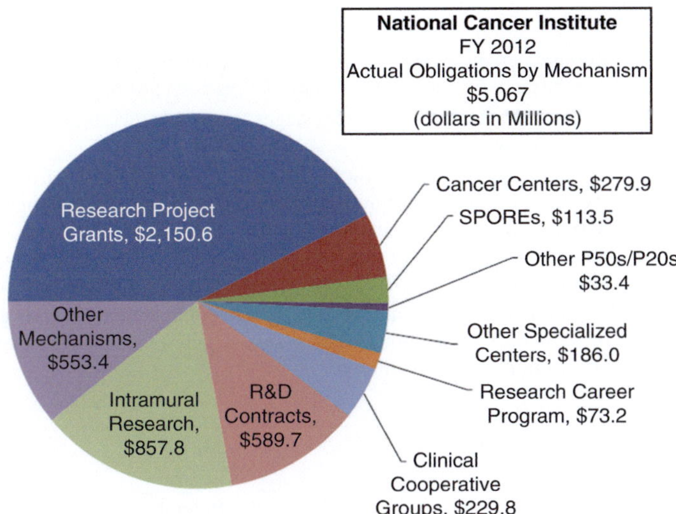

Fig. 8.5 NCI grant disbursements. More than two billion dollars per year is disbursed through NCI extramural grants [72]

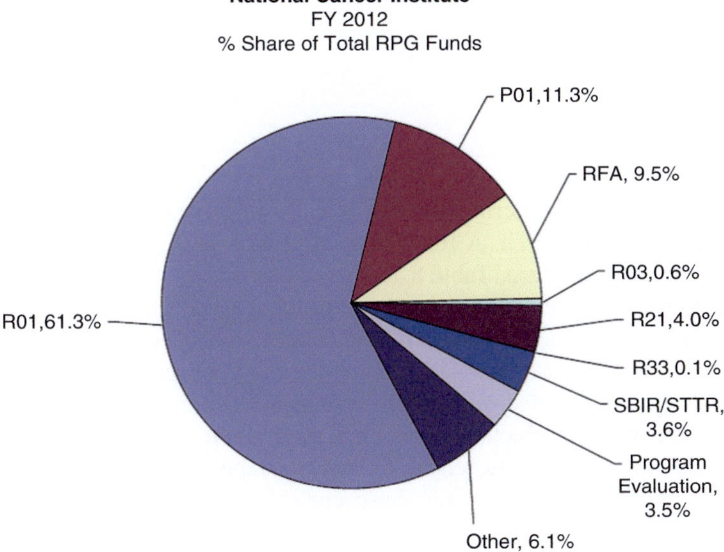

Fig. 8.6 NCI grants disbursed by type. Most extramural grants fall into the research grant category (*R01*), or project grant category (*PO1*) [72]

Table 8.7 Grant categories

R series	Research grants. These include the most common type of grant, the R01, which is a 3–5-year grant for a specific research project
K series	Training grants that span career stages from early investigator towards independence in research
T& F series	Research and training fellowships aimed at institutions (T) or individuals (F). Most of the F series awards, the Ruth L. Kirschstein National Research Service Awards, are limited to US citizens, non-citizen nationals or lawfully admitted US permanent residents. However, non-NRSA fellowships are available through the NIH Fogarty International Center (see below)
P series	Program or Project Center Grants. Typically larger than R-series grants, these include among others, P01 grants, which address integrated multi-project funding for institutions

Table 8.8 Funding per country 2013

Australia	$564,591
Belarus	$95,313
Belgium	$287,528
Canada	$6,924,677
Costa Rica	$2,280,313
France	$2,544,098
India	$183,930
Israel	$1,119,051
Korea, Republic of	$160,786
Netherlands	$204,335
Sweden	$44,712
UK	$4,292,430
	$18,701,764

The NCI offers a bewildering array of grants—understanding the nomenclature itself requires some research. A full listing of grant types is available online [73], but briefly the categories are (Table 8.7):

The investigator may also come across funding types that are not grants; the common ones are contract mechanisms and cooperative agreements. Briefly, a contract like an "N01" is just that—a formal agreement between NCI and a research institution for provision of specified deliverables in a certain timeframe. A cooperative agreement funding mechanism is employed when substantial programmatic involvement is anticipated between the NCI and the recipient institution. Cooperative agreements require that both parties have close, ongoing contact and make decisions together.

NCI can award grants directly to foreign institutions, but a review of fiscal year 2013 (FY2013) expenditures shows that little of this funding was directed to LMIC institutions. According to the FY 2013 DEA Annual Report [74], the only low- or lower-middle-income country to receive direct funding was India for an R01 project on Early Detection of Common Cancers in Women (Table 8.8).

However, this does not tell the whole story, as most of the funding directed towards LMICs is provided as foreign components of domestic research grants and

Table 8.9 FY2013 NCI domestic awards with an LMIC foreign component

Funding mechanism	Number awarded	Description	Funding amount
D43	8	International Research Training Grants to support research training programs for US and foreign professionals and students to strengthen global health research and international research collaboration	$1,858,152
F30	1	Pre-doctoral national research service award: Individual fellowships for pre-doctoral training which leads to the combined M.D./Ph.D. degrees	$46,107
F32	2	Postdoctoral Individual National Research Service Award to provide postdoctoral research training to individuals to broaden their scientific background and extend their potential for research in specified health-related areas	$106,132
K05	1	Support for a research scientist qualified to pursue independent research which would extend the research program of the sponsoring institution, or to direct an essential part of this research program	$172,582
K23	1	Mentored Patient-Oriented Research Career Development Award to provide support for the career development of investigators who have made a commitment to patient-oriented research. This mechanism provides support for a 3-year minimum up to 5-year period of supervised study and research for clinically trained professionals who have the potential to develop into productive, clinical investigators	$142,429
R01	17	Research Project Grant	$8,132,674
R03	2	Small Research Project Grant	$152,726
R21	2	Exploratory/Developmental Research Project Grant	$410,980
U01	1	Clinical Research Cooperative Agreement	$12,077,537
U24	1	Cooperative agreement for resource-related research projects	$2,346,388
			$25,445,707

US National Cancer Institute (2014) 2013 Division of Extramural Affairs Annual Report

contracts. Some of these funding resources underwrite direct cooperation between US and overseas institutions; while others focus on training as part of institutional capacity building or "twinning" programs between US and foreign institutions (Tables 8.9, 8.10, 8.11 and 8.12).

In addition to considering NCI in terms of funding mechanisms, several programs within NCI are relevant for cancer research and clinical trials outside the US.

The Cancer Therapy Evaluation Program (*CTEP*): This program within the NCI Division of Cancer Treatment and Diagnosis oversees clinical trials in the National Clinical Trial Network, a predominantly North American network comprising more

Table 8.10 FY2013 NCI domestic awards with an LMIC component by funding mechanism

Funding Mechanism

Country	D43	F30	F32	K05	K23	R01	R03	R21	U01	U24	Sub-total
Bangladesh						3					3
Benin						1					1
Cameroon	1					1					2
Egypt						3				1	4
Honduras							1				1
India			1	1		4	1			1	8
Kenya	1	1				2			1		5
Malawi						1		1			2
Nicaragua							1				1
Nigeria	1		1					1			3
Pakistan										1	1
Rwanda	1										1
Tanzania	1					1					2
Uganda	2				1	3			1		7
Vietnam						1					1
Zambia	1					2					3
Zimbabwe									1		1

US National Cancer Institute (2014) 2013 Division of Extramural Affairs Annual Report

Table 8.11 Amount allocated to LMIC foreign components within NCI domestic awards in FY 2013

Country	Multiple country grant	Single country grant
Bangladesh	$2,473,244	$1,957,950
Benin	$348,000	
Cameroon	$348,000	
Egypt	$3,305,184	$958,796
Honduras	$78,000	
India	$4,328,634	$1,457,697
Kenya	$12,996,600	$571,063
Malawi	$378,037	$378,037
Nicaragua	$78,000	
Nigeria	$537,396	$483,454
Pakistan	$2,346,388	
Rwanda	$233,329	$233,329
Tanzania	$233,333	
Uganda	$14,054,020	$1,628,483
Vietnam	$618,947	$618,947
Zambia	$1,095,576	$747,576
Zimbabwe	$12,077,537	

Note: A large part of the sum in the multi-country grant column for Kenya, Uganda, South Africa, and Zimbabwe comes from a $12,077,537 U01 grant from the NCI Office for HIV and AIDS Malignancies to the AIDS Malignancy Consortium sites in these countries

US National Cancer Institute (2014) 2013 Division of Extramural Affairs Annual Report

Table 8.12 FY2013 NCI domestic awards with a foreign component in an LMIC by thematic category

Category	Countries
AIDS Cancer	Kenya (2), Malawi, Rwanda, Tanzania, Uganda (4), Zambia, Zimbabwe
Applied Cancer Screening Research	India (2)
Biochemistry and Pharmacology	India (2)
Cancer Disparities	Uganda
Cancer Etiology	Kenya, Malawi
Chemoprevention	Bangladesh (2)
Clinical Oncology	Egypt, Pakistan
Early Detection: Biomarkers	Egypt
Epidemiology: Host Susceptibility Factors	Egypt
Epidemiology: Modifiable Risk Factors	Egypt, Honduras, Nicaragua, Zambia
Tobacco control	Bangladesh, Benin, Cameroon, India, Kenya, Uganda, Vietnam, Zambia
Training	India (2), Kenya, Uganda

US National Cancer Institute (2014) 2013 Division of Extramural Affairs Annual Report

than 3,000 hospitals. The network focuses on practice-changing, late-phase cancer treatment trials. Administratively, four US (ALLIANCE, ECOG-ACRIN, NRG, and SWOG) and one Canadian-based (NCIC-CTG) cooperative groups conduct clinical trials in adults, in addition to the US-based Children's Oncology Group (COG) dedicated to pediatric trials. These groups can cooperate with foreign clinical research centers or foreign networks to conduct clinical trials, although the process is complex [75] and tends to be reserved for trials with high scientific priority that cannot be conducted within the North American networks alone.

Some of the NCTN Groups have developed relationships with overseas sites, such that NCTN studies are available to these sites (pending logistical and regulatory issues, such as drug availability at the foreign site). These sites benefit not only from the clinical trial infrastructure of the NCTN groups, but compensation for accrual on a per patient basis. Presently, almost all of these sites are located in countries classified as upper-middle or high income; the exceptions in a recent survey were lower-middle income sites in Egypt and India. LMIC clinical investigators interested in collaborating with the NCTN, whether to lead or cooperate in an international trial, should contact a disease subject expert within one of the cooperative groups (Table 8.13).

Another office within CTEP, the Investigatory Drugs Branch, oversees early phase clinical trials; these are more often conducted by single institutions or consortia. This office accepts unsolicited letters of intent for clinical trials involving drugs within their development portfolio. An investigator from an LMIC would need to make a strong case that the study needs to be conducted in their region either due to specific expertise or some other comparative advantage such as high prevalence of an uncommon cancer. At the same time, it would be necessary to provide assurances

Table 8.13 Global sites eligible to enroll patients on NCTN trials as of March 2014

		Adult				Pediatric
		ALLIANCE	ECOG-ACRIN	NRG	SWOG	COG
Argentina	Upper-middle	1				1
Australia	High		1	2		8
Brazil	Upper-middle		1			3
Chile	High					1
China	Upper-middle		1	1		
Columbia	Upper-middle				1	
Egypt	Lower-middle					1
Germany	High		2			
Hong Kong	High			3		
India	Lower-middle			1		2
Ireland	High	1	17	20		1
Israel	High		2	4		1
Italy	High			1		
Japan	High		5	18		
Mexico	Upper-middle	1			1	1
Netherlands	High			1		1
New Zealand	High					2
Peru	Upper-middle		2		1	
Poland	High			2		
Saudi Arabia	High			1	1	1
Singapore	High			1		
South Africa	Upper-middle		1			
South Korea	High		11	15	1	
Spain	High		20	7	20	
Switzerland	High			1		3
Taiwan	n/a			1		
UAE	High			1		
UK	High			3		

regarding quality of the staff and site to conduct the trial. The same office can also make small amounts of investigational agents available internationally for preclinical studies, which may benefit researchers who need the drug to generate preliminary data that could support the later submission of a clinical trial concept. The list of drugs in the CTEP portfolio is available online [76], as are the guidelines and forms for submission of a letter of intent [77].

Office of HIV/AIDS and HIV Malignancies (OHAM): In the last decade, much of the US government research funding for LMICs has been dedicated to HIV/AIDS. As reflected in the NCI project listings above, collaborators in LMICs have been awarded funding for a number of projects in AIDS-related malignancies. The NCI

Table 8.14 Other sources of NCI extramural funding

NCI organization	Mission
Division of Cancer Biology[a]	Basic research in all areas of cancer biology
Division of Cancer Control and Population Sciences[a]	Research in surveillance, epidemiology, health services, behavioral science, and cancer survivorship. Of particular interest to LMIC researchers, DCCPS is responsible for programs in implementation science
Division of Cancer Prevention[a]	Research to determine a person's risk of developing cancer and to find ways to reduce that risk. This includes clinical trials in cancer prevention
Division of Cancer Treatment and Diagnosis[a]	This division pursues prospective leads in cancer detection and treatment (new agents, biomarkers, imaging tests, radiation, surgery, and immunotherapy) and advances them towards application. This includes interventional clinical trials
Center for Strategic Scientific Initiatives[a]	This office implements exploratory and transdisciplinary studies. The offices of nanotechnology and proteomics are within this center
Center to Reduce Cancer Health Disparities[a]	Health disparities research and training
Office of Cancer Centers[a]	NCI-designated cancer centers are national centers of clinical and research excellence
	This is a domestic program. However, many of the cancer centers participate in projects or maintain twinning arrangements with sister institutions in LMICs. Contact the NCI Center for Global Health (NCIGlobalHealth@mail.nih.gov) for updated information regarding cancer center collaborations in individual LMICs
Office of Cancer Complementary and Alternative Medicines[a]	Research on identifying novel therapeutics from traditional treatments, complementary approaches to cancer therapy, lifestyle modifications, and cancer outcomes

[a]US National Cancer Institute (2014) 2013 Division of Extramural Affairs Annual Report

Office of HIV and AIDS Malignancy spearheads this effort. A list of funding opportunities for cancer research in the context of HIV/AIDS is kept up-to-date on the OHAM website [78].

This office also oversees the AIDS Malignancy Consortium, a clinical trial network involving both cancer centers in the US, South Africa, Kenya, Uganda, and Zimbabwe. Investigators interested in possible collaboration with this network may wish to contact the program through its website [79].

Other sources of extramural funding within NCI include the following (Table 8.14):

The Center for Global Health (CGH) was established in 2011 at the NCI to help reduce the global burden of cancer. CGH develops initiatives and collaborates with other NCI divisions, NCI-designated cancer centers, and countries to support cancer control planning, build capacity, and support cancer research and cancer research networks in LMICs.

CGH Short-Term Scientist Exchange Program (STSEP)

This program promotes exchanges in either direction between US and foreign laboratory scientists from low-, low-middle-, and upper-middle-income countries. The duration of these exchanges is limited to 6 months. Applications are accepted throughout the year, with funding decisions taken quarterly. Applicants must be proficient in English, have a Ph.D., M.D., or equivalent degree, at least 1 year of postdoctoral experience, and have an invitation from a qualified host organization [80].

Low-Cost Technology for Health Research in LMICs Grants

In 2013, the NCI Center for Global Health created a funding opportunity to support the development of low-cost technologies for cancer detection, diagnosis, and treatment, with intended application in LMICs (RF-CA-13-015: Cancer Detection, Diagnosis, and Treatment Technologies for Global Health [81]). In the first year of this program, NCI funded six projects and the National Institute for Biomedical Imaging and Bioengineering supported another two. Funding of up to $500,000 per year was available in the exploratory phase (up to 2 years) and up to $1,000,000 per year for the validation phase (up to 3 years). NCI has indicated the intention to continue this program in the future [82].

BIG Cat Grants

The Center has also provided funding for the Beginning Investigator Grant for Catalytic Research (BIG Cat) program, which supports exploratory data collection by African scientists performing cancer research in Africa; investigators outside Africa are not eligible, although collaboration with African investigators is encouraged. The program is entirely administered by AORTIC, the African Organisation for Research and Training in Cancer. Thus far, there have been two BIG Cat cohorts, each with six awardees. Each awardee received $25,000 per year for a 2-year period. Investigators interested in this funding source are advised to monitor the AORTIC website for publication of letter of intent instructions, which detail the application process. In the past, the application process was supervised by AORTIC Operations Manager Belmira Rodrigues, aortic@telkomsa.net.

The NCI Summer Curriculum in Cancer Prevention

Every year, NCI hosts a summer curriculum in cancer prevention open to both domestic and international physicians, scientists, and healthcare professions who have an interest in cancer prevention and control. The curriculum spans July and

August, consisting of a 4-week Principles and Practices in Cancer Prevention and Control Course, a 1-week course in Molecular Prevention, and the Annual Advances in Cancer Prevention Lecture. The curriculum is overseen by researchers from the NCI Division of Cancer Prevention, but faculty for the courses is drawn from all parts of NCI, other government agencies, academic institutions, cancer centers, and public and private organizations. It is recommended that participants in the course have backgrounds in epidemiology, biostatistics, and cancer biology; preference is given to individuals with a doctor degree.

The course involves no tuition or other material costs. The NCI Center for Global Health provides funding to cover living expenses and, in some cases, travel expenses for a limited number of applicants from low- and middle-income countries. Since 2006, between 25 and 45 participants from LMICs have taken part each year. Information about the program, past course syllabi, and application details are available online [83].

Grant Writing Workshops

The CGH has led efforts to develop grant-writing skills among researchers in Latin America, Sub-Saharan Africa, and the Caribbean. These workshops have included the participation not only of NCI but also several other NIH institutes and centers, the WHO, PAHO, WHO/AFRO, Wellcome Trust (UK), CDC, USAID, IARC, UICC as well as local partners including the Colombian Ministry of Health, the SAMRC, and the Caribbean Public Health Agency. Future workshops will be announced online [84].

The NIH Fogarty International Center (FIC: While many of the centers and institutes at the NIH are engaged in global health research as part of their overall mission, global health is the central mission of the FIC. The center's remit includes formulation of high-level global health policy, establishment of international institutional partnerships, and of particular relevance to cancer researchers in LMICs, supporting international scientific collaboration and training. The Center's FY2014 budget justification requested total funds of almost $73 million to perform these activities [85].

FIC supports basic, clinical, and applied research and training for US and foreign investigators working in the developing world. Since its formation more than 40 years ago, Fogarty has served as a bridge between NIH and the greater global health community: facilitating exchanges among investigators, providing training opportunities, and supporting promising research initiatives in developing countries. Over the last four decades, about 5,000 scientists worldwide have received significant research training through Fogarty Programs.

Currently, Fogarty funds some 400 research and training projects involving more than 100 US universities. The US scientists, in turn, collaborate with colleagues in many countries, most of them in LMICs. Fogarty also convenes the best scientific minds around the world to address critical global health research problems such as polio eradication, the impact of climate change on disease outbreaks, and strengthening research capacity in LMICs.

A full listing of the center's funding opportunities targeted to LMICs is available online, but a few key programs with particular relevance to cancer researcher are highlighted below (Table 8.15).

These programs are aimed primarily at investigators and institutions in LMICs, but the Fogarty Center also supports several programs to give US investigators experience working with LMIC institutions (Table 8.16):

Other NIH institutes are also active in many LMICs. The National Institute for Allergy and Infectious Diseases (NIAID) has projects worldwide addressing infectious disease; about two million cancers a year are attributable to infectious etiologies, particularly in LMICs [86]. Similarly, institutes that concentrate on specific organ systems have a stake in cancer research, for example the National Heart, Lung, and Blood Institute has strong interest in lung cancer, leukemia, and transplant medicine. The National Institute of Diabetes and Digestive and Kidney Diseases (NIDDK) conducts research on obesity, behavior, and metabolism in connection with carcinogenesis, particularly of pancreatic cancer. Some institutes such as the National Human Genome Research Institutes (NHGRI) oversee research that cuts across disease fields. For example, the NHGRI's Ethical, Legal and Social Implications (ELSI) program could be of interest to cancer researchers looking at gene polymorphisms in a population or performing precision medicine trials with targeted agents [87]. Funding announcements by NCI [88], these other NIH institutes (NIAID [89], NHLBI [90], NIDDK [91], NHGRI [92]), and by the NIH at large [93] are published on their respective websites.

The United States Agency for International Development

Within the US Government, United States Agency for International Development (USAID) takes the lead on foreign assistance, working in many sectors including health. The US Global Development Lab within USAID coordinates the Partnerships for Enhanced Engagement in Research Program, PEER [94]. This is a competitive grants program that invites scientists from developing countries to apply for funding for research and capacity building. PEER involves cooperation of the US National Academy of Sciences as a reviewing body and other US Government Agency Partners including the NIH. Awardees must already be the principal investigator or co-principal investigator supported by an active research award from a US government agency. Supported activities under the PEER award include LMIC research projects, application of new or existing methodologies, practices or protocols in a developing country setting, data collection, and exchange. Certain activities are excluded, such as randomized clinical trials and training programs, workshops, and conferences not directly tied to a research project. Research projects must be led by an LMIC investigator, be primarily carried out in an LMIC, and advance the development of that LMIC.

Table 8.15 Key programs relevant to cancer researchers

International Cooperative Biodiversity Groups[a]	These cooperative agreements involve both US-based researchers and LMIC counterparts exploring health applications for biodiversity research, for example drug discovery. Beyond laboratory research, the intent of this funding is to invest in research capacity to support sustainable and equitable use of these natural resources
Chronic, Non-Communicable Diseases and Disorders Across the Lifespan: Fogarty International Research Training Award[a]	The goal of this program is to sustainably strengthen the research capacity of LMIC institutions and to train their staff to conduct research on chronic, non-communicable diseases and disorders, with the goal of implementing locally appropriate evidence-based public health measures. Cancer is specifically included within the scope of this award
Global Health Research and Training eCapacity Initiative[a]	Applicants at LMIC institutions who have been PIs or collaborators on previous Fogarty grants are eligible for this grant, which supports incorporation of Information and Communication Technology (ICT) into global health research and training
Informatics Training for Global Health[a]	This award provides up to 5 years of funding for researchers at LMIC institutions partnered with US institutions and investigators to develop informatics capacity and support research
Global Health Initiative for New Foreign Investigators[a]	This grant supports career development LMIC researchers who have trained abroad, but then return to their home countries. The intention is to retain these researchers in their home countries where they can share their expertise
Fogarty International Research Collaboration Award[a]	A number of NIH institutes and centers cosponsor this award, which benefits both NIH-supported scientists in the US and their research collaborators in LMICs
Framework Programs for Global Health Innovation (FRAME Innovation)[a]	Support for both US and LMIC institutions to develop broadly interdisciplinary, postdoctoral (or post-terminal degree) research training programs in global health directed towards encouraging innovation in health-related products, processes, and policies. The program emphasizes hands-on, problem-solving, and collaborative approaches and allows US and LMIC trainees to be trained together
International Tobacco and Health Research and Capacity Building Program[a]	This grant is awarded to research institutions in LMICS with the intention of institutional capacity building and promoting tran-disciplinary research aimed at reducing the global burden of morbidity and mortality caused by tobacco use
International Research Ethics Education and Curriculum Development Award[a]	This award funds development of a masters-level curriculum in bioethics by research institutions in LMICs
Medical Partnership Initiative (MEPI)[a]	This award is available only to LMIC institutions that have previously received support from PEPFAR and PEPFAR partners to develop and improve medical education. While this program is targeted at HIV rather than cancer, many of the same institutions providing HIV care are also leading institutions for cancer care and research

[a]US National Cancer Institute (2014) 2013 Division of Extramural Affairs Annual Report

Table 8.16 Programs for US researchers working with LMIC institutions

International Research Scientist Development Award[a]	Applicants must be US citizens with a doctoral-level degree in a research or health-related field. The awardee must spend at least 50 % of their time in an LMIC institution and have both LMIC and US-based mentors
Fulbright-Fogarty Fellows in Public Health[a]	This is limited to medical and graduate students who are US citizens and who will conduct research projects in an eligible LMIC country (see the list: http://us.fulbrightonline.org/fulbright-fogarty-fellowships-in-public-health)
Fulbright-Fogarty Scholars in Public Health[a]	This is limited to postdoctoral students in public health research who are US citizens and who will conduct research at a Fogarty-affiliated site in specific LMIC (refer to the annual program announcement: http://www.cies.org/program/fulbright-fogarty-postdoctoral-awards)

[a]US National Cancer Institute (2014) 2013 Division of Extramural Affairs Annual Report

Since its launch in 2011, this funding mechanism has supported more than 150 projects in 40 countries, an investment of about $28 million. Forty-six projects were launched in 2014 to advance the scientific and technical capacity of both the US and partner countries in critical areas of development. These projects span such diverse research areas as maternal and child health, glacier retreat and water resource sustainability, biodiversity conservation, biogas production, drought and climate change mitigation, and pollution remediation.

Not every topic fits within the PEER framework—the topic must align with USAID objectives. There are global, regional, and country-specific calls for proposals across all research sectors [95]. For the most part, these calls have not been cancer-specific, but investigators have successfully embedded cancer control research within broader developmental topics. For example, tobacco control research is part of both the Philippine and Indonesian PEER programs. In the Philippines, it was embedded within a tuberculosis project entitled "Effect of a smoking cessation intervention program for families of children diagnosed with tuberculosis" conducted by researchers from the Philippine Ambulatory Pediatric Association in partnership with investigators from Massachusetts General Hospital and Harvard Medical School. In Indonesia, the project came under the heading of maternal-child health, "Examining the Effects of air pollution in early life on infant and maternal health" conducted by researchers from Cipto Mangunkusumo National General Hospital and the Kerstin Klipstein-Grobusch University Medical Center in the US.

Investigators interested in this funding mechanism should review USAID country development priorities prior to preparing an application. These priorities are stated on country-specific USAID mission websites and Country Development Cooperation Strategy (CDCS) documents [96]. Investigators should then contact the USAID mission in their country to discuss how their research would dovetail with local USAID development priorities. Applications for the PEER program are made online [97].

Table 8.17 Pasteur Institute Network locations in low- and lower-middle-income countries

Bangui, Central African Republic	Low
Antananarivo, Madagascar	Low
Phnom Penh, Cambodia	Low
Yaounde, Cameroon	Lower-middle
Abidjan, Côte d'Ivoire	Lower-middle
Casablanca, Morocco	Lower-middle
Dakar, Senegal	Lower-middle
Vientiane, Laos	Lower-middle
Hanoi, Vietnam	Lower-middle
Ho Chi Minh City, Vietnam	Lower-middle
Nha Trang, Vietnam	Lower-middle

International Organizations

Institut Pasteur

The Institut Pasteur is a private, state-approved foundation based in France with an annual operating budget of 270.5€ million in 2012. Its threefold mission comprises research, public health, and teaching, but what sets the institute apart is its international network consisting of 32 institutes. The institute does not award grants, but funds research and training within its network. For those investigators who reside in a country where the institute has a presence, a logical first step would be to look into the personnel and projects already under way in the national institution and to try to find a good match in terms of research interests. The Institute provides research support and training at various levels of career advancement for applicants from France, but also for foreign researchers within the Institut Pasteur International Network (RIIP). A full listing of open applications for traineeships, doctoral, postdoctoral programs, study, and conference grants is available on the website [98]. The institute offers a wide array of courses worldwide through its network including locations in LMICs; many of the courses, for example instruction in biostatistics and data analysis, have direct application to cancer research [99] (Table 8.17).

Multilateral Banks

World Bank

The World Bank Institute administers two scholarship programs that enable graduate students from developing countries to study abroad. The McNamara Scholarship provides for a 5- to 10-month visit to a foreign institution, whereas the joint Japanese/World Bank Scholarship Program enables mid-career professionals to live and study abroad for longer periods. Since these programs are not restricted by area of study, students from LMICs interested in any aspect of cancer research could consider these scholarships [100].

Islamic Development Bank

The Islamic Development Bank (IDB) funds scholarships in science and technology fields. These are offered to candidates pursuing studies in science, technology, and medicine in specified countries. A Master of Science scholarship allows students to study in their home countries, whereas an advanced scholarship provides up to 3 years of doctoral funding and up to a year of postdoctoral funding at recognized international institutions. In the latter case, recipients are required to agree to return to their country of origin after studies are complete [101].

The World Academy of Sciences

TWAS was founded in 1983 in Trieste, Italy, with core support from the Italian government and is now a program unit within the United Nations Educational, Scientific, and Cultural Organization (UNESCO). TWAS maintains regional offices in Brazil, Egypt, Kenya, India, and China. The overall emphasis on TWAS is building capacity of researchers in LMICs and in promoting South–South cooperation. In 2013, total organizational expenditures amounted to about $5.6 million [102].

Calls for funding run the gamut of scientific inquiry, but tend towards more basic science. To give a sense of funding levels, in 2013, 44 TWAS research grants for individuals were awarded in amounts of up to $15,000 each and 20 TWAS research grants for groups were awarded in amounts of up to $30,000 each [102]. A listing of current research grants, doctoral and postdoctoral fellowships, funding for scientific meetings, and opportunities for scientists to visit developing nations can be found on their website [103].

Union for International Cancer Control

The Union for International Cancer Control (UICC) is a membership organization founded in 1933 and based in Geneva. Its goal is to help the global community accelerate the fight against cancer, and it is well placed to do, with membership across 155 countries and partners including international organizations, ministries of health, research institutes, major cancer societies, and cancer advocacy groups. Fellowships programs are a core activity of UICC and more than 6,000 fellowships have been awarded to date.

The UICC administers the American Cancer Society (ACS) International Fellowship for Beginning Investigators, which provides for a 12-month fellowship for researchers devoted to projects in LMICs. The fellowship supports researchers in epidemiology and cancer control, as well as other cancer research fields, excluding clinical research. The UICC also supports two shorter-term technology transfer fellowships—the 3-month Yamigawa-Yoshida Memorial International Cancer Study Grant and the International Cancer Technology Transfer Fellowship, with 1-month duration. The UICC may at times offer other fellowships, including some with geographical restrictions [104].

United Nations

World Health Organization

When member states of the World Health Organization (WHO) made the pledge to achieve universal coverage in 2005, they effectively launched a research agenda to address the dominant health needs of WHO member states, to support national health research systems, to set norms and standards for the proper conduct of research, and to accelerate the translation of research findings into health policy and practice [105]. The WHO supports basic, applied research, operational (implementation), and translational research in LMICS as well as health policy and systems research [106].

The WHO is not itself a grant-making component of the UN, but it does contribute funding to other programs that fund research such as UNITAID (Innovative Financing to Shape Markets for HIV/AIDS, Malaria and Tuberculosis), and the Tropical Diseases Research program, a joint initiative supported by WHO, the United Nations Development Program (UNDP), and the World Bank, the Global Vaccine (GAVI) Alliance, and the Global Fund to Fight AIDS, Tuberculosis, and Malaria.

International Agency for Research on Cancer

Within WHO, the International Agency for Research on Cancer (IARC) focuses on cancer prevention research. IARC oversees WHO programs in development of cancer registries, biobanks, and information resources and curates scientific evidence to inform global cancer control policies. IARC does not offer project-specific grants, but it does support training for cancer research including fellowships for young scientists, expertise transfer fellowships, and awards for senior visiting scientists. Additionally, the IARC conducts a summer course in epidemiology yearly in Lyon, France. Participation of researchers from LMICs is encouraged in all of these programs; in 2012, 58 % of fellows were from LMICs [107].

Each year, postdoctoral fellowships are offered to about 8–11 young investigators, who are within 5 years of completing their doctoral studies. Research is conducted at the IARC research group in Lyon, France, for a period of up to 2 years and then fellows are expected to return to their home countries. The fellowship covers a number of fields relevant to cancer prevention research including epidemiology, biostatistics, bioinformatics, molecular and cell biology, molecular genetics, epigenetics, and molecular pathology. Fellowships are not awarded in areas of clinical medicine, diagnostics, therapy, or medicinal drugs [108]. The senior visiting scientist fellowship is meant to allow a more established researcher to spend 6–12 months with the IARC research group. Conversely, the expertise transfer fellowship enables an established investigator to spend the same period in a low- or medium-resource country with the objective of transferring specific research expertise and knowledge to researchers in that location.

In addition, each summer, the IARC conducts a summer school for cancer epidemiology. The course is targeted to epidemiologists, statisticians, physicians, oncologists, public health specialists, and others with a direct interest in working in cancer epidemiology or registration. Participants from LMICs are encouraged and are exempt from the course fee. For a limited number of participants, the IARC also provides financial support for travel and accommodation [109]. The IARC and UICC jointly offer a Development Fellowship Award to allow one person from the summer course to return to IARC for 3 months to receive additional training and/or to pursue collaborative research.

Special Programme for Research and Training in Tropical Diseases

The Special Programme for Research and Training in Tropical Diseases (TDR) was established in 1975 by the WHO. The WHO is the implementing agency for this program, which is co-sponsored by other UN agencies including the United Nations Children's Fund (UNICEF), the UNDP, and the World Bank. The program was developed to address infectious diseases of poverty and has traditionally focused on HIV, malaria, tuberculosis, and endemic vector-borne parasitic diseases. As such, the program has relevance to cancer research where there is overlap between these diseases and cancer. The program also addresses research topics, which are equally valuable for cancer research: biotechnology, capacity strengthening, diagnostics, drug discovery, environmental studies, health systems and implementation research, drug and product development, and social and economic research. Grants available through this program are described on the WHO website [110]. In some cases, it may make sense for cancer researchers in LMICs to team up with their infectious disease counterparts to pursue larger projects that could serve both fields. In addition to project grants, the TDR supports training and fellowship opportunities, a proportion of which focus on methodology rather than specific diseases [110].

The Pan American Health Organization

In addition to its global programs, WHO is also organized regionally, with offices covering member states in Africa, the Americas, South-East Asia, Europe, the Eastern Mediterranean, and Western Pacific [111]. The Regional Office for the Americas is best known as PAHO, the Pan American Health Organization. Some of the work that PAHO is doing to support researchers and research infrastructure is detailed below, but researchers in each region would do well to investigate the programs supported by their respective regional offices.

Researchers in Latin America benefit from work PAHO has undertaken in the domains of policy, identification of available and needed resources, and training. PAHO Member States formalized a policy underlining the need for standardization and strengthening of research capacity as a foundation for improving health and advancing development in the region (Resolution CD49.R10 [112]). This policy stresses the need of governance and stewardship within the health sector, the responsibilities of the health sector, and also the value and need for cooperation with other sectors dealing with determinants of health; for example, safe housing, adequate nutrition, healthy habits, tobacco, and exposure to other environmental hazards. As part of the policy implementation, PAHO has mapped regional research capacities and frameworks both overall and specifically for cancer research, the latter in collaboration with the NIH and NCI [113].

Research management is a need (and bottleneck) in many research centers. PAHO has partnered with CIDEIM (Centro Internacional de Entrenamiento e Investigaciones Médicas) [114] to train teams of researchers in the Americas on effective project planning and evaluation. About 400 researchers have been trained under a train-the-trainer scheme that lead to the training of 50 specialized trainers who support the expansion of this program from training centers in Cali (Colombia), Tegucigalpa (Honduras), Bello Horizonte (Brazil), and Kingston (Jamaica) [115].

Finally, PAHO and the Organization of American States (OAS) agreed to launch a scholarship program to promote training in health and health research [116]. The awards cover tuition and a living allowance for work at the masters or doctoral level in health-related fields at Brazilian universities [117].

Charities

A number of charities support cancer research in LMICs; these include large private foundations like the Gates Foundation, Global Fund, and Wellcome Trust with general interests in global health; cancer-specific charities such as the ACS, CRUK, WCRF; and cancer advocacy-based organizations like the Komen Foundation.

American Cancer Society

The ACS is a US-based not-for-profit organization that provides extensive programs and services for cancer patients and the public. Additionally, it administers both intramural and extramural research programs. The extramural program encompasses research grants and health professional training awards for nurses, physicians, and oncology social work professionals. Research grants and mentored training and career development grants offered by the organization are restricted to US citizens or permanent residents. Additionally, the organization supports the Beginning Investigators awards through the UICC, as detailed above, which is explicitly aimed at investigators from LMICs.

Bill and Melinda Gates Foundation

Founded at the turn of the century, the Bill and Melinda Gates Foundation is one of the largest private charities in the world, with an endowment of about $40 billion and grant awards of about $3.5 billion in 2013. Both global health and development are core priorities for the foundation. While health funding has largely focused on infectious diseases such as HIV and malaria in the last decade, programs promoting vaccination have also contributed to cancer control. Similarly, global tobacco is a strategic priority, which the foundation approaches through policy work and social marketing, but also funding for global and locally-based research to inform such efforts. While the majority of grants are provided to implementing organizations for direct provision of services and distribution of resources, substantial funding is channeled towards research.

Some funding awards are made with specific grantees in mind, others are open calls with defined priorities. Unsolicited proposals are not accepted. Grants are awarded to organizations, not individuals [118].

Two categories of grant may be of particular interest to cancer researchers. The first is the Grand Challenges Grant, a standing program to find innovative solutions to specific global problems. The philosophy behind this program is that major advances may require investment in projects that are too risky for other donors. If funded pilots prove their worth, the foundation may provide follow-on funding. For researchers, an attractive aspect of these grants is that they require less preliminary data than many other programs [119]. Additionally, the foundation reviews concept memos for global health grants in targeted areas on a continual basis [120]. Aside from funding research projects, the foundation has funded conferences to bring together researchers to address LMIC cancer research issues.

Cancer Research UK

Cancer Research UK (CRUK) is a UK-based charity, which in 2013/2014 disbursed £351 million to research institutions, hospitals, and universities across the UK [121]. A number of CRUK-sponsored projects are international in scope; funding is provided to a UK-based host institution, which then manages the grant reward and is responsible for the flow of funds to researchers outside the UK. Some examples in the current portfolio include assessments of HPV versus cytological testing conducted in Mexico and Costa Rica; a study of environmental risk factors for esophageal cancer in Iran; a study of adjuvant aspirin therapy involving sites in India; and, the CONCORD-2 project involving data from 160 cancer registries in 50 countries. LMIC researchers interested in applying will need a UK-based partner, who can then follow the standard procedures to apply through a response mode funding committee. In addition, CRUK supports a number of career development awards, which may be relevant for UK-based researchers who study cancer in LMICs or related topics such as tobacco control [122].

Global Fund to Fight AIDS, Tuberculosis, and Malaria

It seems counterintuitive to look for cancer research funding from an organization that defines itself by three diseases that are not cancer, but there are basic and clinical science questions that involve both cancer and these diseases. Certainly, there are AIDS-related cancers, most prominently Kaposi sarcoma and AIDS-related lymphoma. Similarly, there is the association of Burkitt Lymphoma and malaria. In all three diseases, as in cancer, evasion of immune clearance is a key mechanism undermining treatment effectiveness. Similarly, healthcare strengthening efforts aimed at fighting these infectious diseases will benefit cancer care and vice versa. Likewise, implementation research aimed at assessing these interventions could easily serve the intent of both this fund and the cancer researcher.

Much of the fund goes directly into provision of medical care and resources such as health products and pharmaceuticals (21 %), medicines and pharmaceutical products (19 %), and the human resources, program management, and training necessary to keep programs operation [123]; however, some funding expended by operational partners is dedicated to research. The majority of Global Fund grants are provided above the level of the individual researcher; the largest recipients are government ministries of health (39 %). However, NGOs, community-based organizations, and academia constitute the next largest bloc (30 %). Given the sheer magnitude of Global Fund spending, even a small fraction of annual spending (overall disbursement of $3.9 billion in 2013) is significant [123].

The website provides only a very high-level view of the project, although researchers may examine the "Grants in Detail" spreadsheet, which does not drill down to project-level detail, but does identify which organization is operationally responsible for AIDS, TB, Malaria, or Health Care Strengthening activities in a given country (the principal recipient) as well as the local funding agency. This information may be helpful in setting up initial contacts to discuss cancer research projects that border on the fund's principal concerns. Finally, both active and expired grants within a national portfolio can be found through the fund's portfolio portal [124].

Susan G. Komen Breast Cancer Foundation

This foundation is a US-based, not-for-profit organization that directly supports breast cancer patients and contributes to research, advocacy, and awareness efforts for that disease. The organization has worldwide reach through its own regional chapters and through numerous partnerships. International grants are awarded by organization and some grants are operational rather than research-oriented, for example community grants to raise awareness, perform community education, implement screening programs, and improve access to care or to train healthcare workers. Other grants do have a research question, often involving epidemiology or implementation science. The foundation does not generally accept unsolicited proposals; rather, calls for proposals are listed regionally on their website [125].

In addition, the foundation provides several categories of grants that support research or research career development. Total outlays to research fund recipients in FY2013 totaled about $37.8 million [126]. For individuals, there are grants for graduate training in disparities research, postdoctoral fellowships, early career development (career catalyst research grants), and investigator-initiated research grants. For multi-disciplinary teams working on projects in emphasis areas defined yearly by the foundation, there are promise grants [127].

According to the foundation's map of research grants distributed worldwide since 1982 [128], no grants have been awarded to investigators in low-income countries, and one has been awarded to a recipient in an LMIC, India. Upper-middle income countries have seen a few grants over these three decades: three in Mexico, three in Brazil, and five in Argentina. The remaining grants have been awarded to investigators in high-income countries, particularly the US. Reviewing funded research reports from FY12 and FY13, no grants were made to recipients in LMICs. However, in FY13 a $967,000 grant was awarded to the WHO's IARC based in France, for a project titled "African Breast Cancer Research Network—Disparities in Outcomes."

Wellcome Trust

The Wellcome Trust is a UK-based global charitable foundation that spends about £600 million every year in the UK and internationally to advance worldwide health. The foundation traces its roots to the drug company founded by Sir Henry Wellcome; however, the industry relationship went in one direction with various mergers with Glaxo and later SmithKlineBeecham to yield GlaxoSmithKline (GSK), while the Trust maintained an independent, non-commercial identity. The trust now focuses on five research challenges, including chronic diseases. The chronic diseases challenge area has been the best funded in recent years [129], and according to the 2010–2020 Strategic Plan [130], explicitly includes cancer. Two other challenge areas, infectious disease and environment, health, and nutrition, may also overlap with cancer research.

Under its international strategy, the Trust funds public health research including early, mid, and late-career fellowships for researchers in LMICs [131]. Initiatives aimed at LMICs may evolve over time and it is best to check the current listing [132], but current funding opportunities are listed in Table 8.18.

In addition, the Trust supports programs directed at specific countries [133]. India is a special case; while all of the above applies to researchers in India, there is also an independent Indian Alliance, an £80 million initiative jointly funded by the Wellcome Trust and the Department of Biotechnology under the Indian MoST. This initiative aims at strengthening the capacity of the Indian scientific community and offers its own fellowships directed at basic, clinical, and public health researchers [134].

World Cancer Research Fund

The World Cancer Research Fund (WCRF) is a London-based, not-for-profit organization with network member organizations in the US, UK, Netherlands, and Hong Kong. Of these, the US-based American Institute for Cancer Research (AICR) seems to be the most active in promoting research in LMICs. The WCRF funds research in cancer prevention, particularly etiologic linkages with diet and physical activity. Investigators bridging developmental work in areas involving food security, lifestyle and cardiovascular risk, epidemiology or metabolomics may find a good match within their calls for funding, which are announced annually [135]. In the

Table 8.18 Current Wellcome Trust funding opportunities

Initiative	Objective	Funding
DELTAS: Developing Excellence in Leadership, Training and Science[a]	An African-led effort to develop a critical mass of internationally competitive researchers working across Africa	Funding for up to 5 years is institutional in nature, covering program administration, grants, awards, training, meetings, research support costs, M&E, research infrastructure, and equipment
Global Health Trials[a]	Support for late-stage (effectively, phase III/IV) interventional clinical trials in LMICs. The most recent call emphasizes chronic NCDs	This is a recurring program collaboratively funded by the Trust, UK MRC, and UK DFID at £15 million per year
Heath Systems Research[a]	To support research to improve health systems in LMICs	This is a recurring program collaboratively funded by the Trust, UK MRC, and UK DFID at £15 million over 3 years

US National Cancer Institute (2014) 2013 Division of Extramural Affairs Annual Report most recent call for funding, applications for investigators in the Americas and Caribbean were directed to the AICR while investigators from all other regions are welcomed, with encouragement for those applying from LMICs.

Pharmaceutical Industry

Several pharmaceutical companies, either directly or through associated foundations, support cancer research through institutional grants, educational activities, and grants for investigator-initiated studies. However, almost all of these efforts are directed at well-resourced countries.

GlaxoSmithKline

GSK have created two regional funding initiatives directed towards health researchers in Latin America and Africa. Trust in Science LATAM was created in 2011 and supports research project funding through a matching fund partnership with government agencies such as the National Brazilian Council of Science and Technology (CNPQ) and Sao Paulo State Foundation for Research Support (FAPESP) in Brazil and the MoST in Argentina. Cancer is not a key research area, although related topics including immunology and inflammation and treatment of some cancer-associated viruses are included. Funding applications are made through partner organizations [136]. Proposals are evaluated jointly by these partners and GSK through independent academic referees. A similar program, Trust in Science Africa, is a more recent addition and is presently limited to scientists in Kenya, Tanzania, and Uganda. Again, cancer research is not identified as a priority area, but GSK do leave the door open for outstanding proposals outside their specific call for proposals. In Africa, funding is awarded directly by GSK after evaluation by an independent advisory panel [137].

In addition to grant-making activities, GSK have announced a £25 million investment in an R&D Open Lab initiative for research on NCDs in Africa [138] This builds on the success of GSK's Open Lab in Tres Cantos, Spain, which gave independent researchers access to GSK facilities, resources, and knowledge to help them advance their own research projects into diseases of the developing world such as malaria, tuberculosis, and leishmaniasis.

The new R&D Open Lab for NCDs in Africa will see GSK scientists collaborate with research and scientific centers across Africa from its Stevenage R&D facility in the UK to conduct high-quality epidemiological, genetic, and interventional research to increase understanding of NCDs in Africa. An independent scientific governing board will oversee the implementation of NCD research projects within a dynamic and networked open innovation environment.

The open lab aims to improve understanding of NCD variations seen in the Africa setting, which could include, for example, the apparent higher prevalence of treatment-resistant hypertension and aggressive breast cancers in younger women. It is hoped that these insights will inform prevention and treatment strategies and will enable researchers across academia and industry to discover and develop new medicines to address the specific needs of African patients. The initiative bears watching as a potential resource for African investigators in need of laboratory collaboration.

Professional Societies

Some funding for cancer research and training directed to LMICs comes from laboratory and clinical researchers themselves through their professional organizations.

American Association for Cancer Research

The American Association for Cancer Research (AACR) is a US-based, professional association focused on cancer research. Through the not-for-profit AACR Foundation for the Prevention and Cure of Cancer and in conjunction with partner organizations, the AACR offers a number of career development fellowships and basic, clinical, epidemiological, and clinical grants on a competitive basis. However, while the organization has a wide international membership base, promoting cancer research in low-resource settings is not a primary objective and some of funding opportunities are only available to researchers in the US. Since grant offerings change over time, investigators should search the current AACR grant database [139]. Investigators outside the US can use webform to exclude studies that are available only within the US.

American Society for Clinical Oncology

In recent years, American Society for Clinical Oncology (ASCO) has greatly increased its international activities. More than a third of ASCO members practice outside the US and the majority of annual meeting attendees hail from overseas [140]. Through its charity arm, the Conquer Cancer Foundation (formerly, the ASCO Cancer Foundation), ASCO offers a range of grants and awards supporting both training and research projects. A number of grants with "international" in the title are aimed at researchers in LMICs. The International Development and Education Award provides early career oncologists in LMICs with a scientific mentor from within ASCO, enables the recipient to attend an annual meeting, and extends complimentary ASCO membership for 3 years. A similar program is aimed at oncologists interested in palliative care, the International Development, and Education Award in Palliative Care [141].

The International Innovation Grant is a $20,000 grant to support a 1-year research project headed by a PI based in an LMIC. The PI must be an ASCO member to qualify. The grant is awarded to the government agency or not-for-profit organization associated with the PI rather than to the individual. The intent is to support hypothesis-driven research that will advance cancer control in the local context, recognizing that what may be considered standard practice in a high-resource setting may not be optimal in a resource-constrained setting [142].

In partnership with LMIC institutions and with partial support from the US NCI, ASCO periodically conducts International Clinical Trials Workshops. These 2-day workshops, organized in collaboration with national or regional oncology societies, provide training for clinical research teams on best practices for clinical trial implementation. During the workshops, globally accepted standards in the conduct of clinical research are reviewed with a local perspective. The schedule for upcoming workshops is available online [143].

Finally, the ASCO Long-Term International Fellowship (LIFe) award allows early-career researchers to spend a year in the US or Canada working with a mentor on a research project. The award is limited to physicians who have gone through the equivalent of a clinical oncology fellowship, have not previously spent substantial time training in North American, and who have less than 10 years' experience in oncology [144].

Other funding mechanisms are not specifically targeted to researchers from LMICs, but are available worldwide on a competitive basis. For example, both the Young Investigator Award and ASCO Career Development Award requests for proposals contain language specifying that the applicant must be a "physician (M.D., D.O., or international equivalent with explanation) working in any country." These two awards respectively provide research project support for individuals in their last 2 years of subspecialty training or in their first 3 years of a full-time faculty position. The Advanced Clinical Research Award, which targets investigators later in their careers, is also open to international applicants. Based on the global map showing all awards made by the Conquer Cancer [145], it is safe to say that over time a substantial proportion of ASCO awards have benefited researchers from LMICs. A full listing of all funding opportunities is available on the ASCO website [146].

European Society for Medical Oncology

The European Society for Medical Oncology (ESMO) is a Swiss-registered, not-for-profit organization and is roughly the European counterpart to ASCO. ESMO does not sponsor funding activities specifically directed towards researchers from LMICs, but in general, its competitive awards are not restricted by geography. A series of fellowship opportunities are offered, from 6-week clinical rotations to translational research placements for up to 2 years [147]. Fellowships cover translational, clinical, and palliative cancer research topics. All the fellowships require that the awardee undergo training at a host institution. ESMO provides a list of institutions willing to host ESMO fellows, but applicants are not restricted to this list. Candidates must be members of ESMO, and it is encouraged that supervisors at both host and originating institution be ESMO members as well. In addition to its own fellowships, ESMO maintains a list of external fellowship opportunities on its website [148].

Clinical Research Workshops

ASCO, AACR, ESMO, and other sponsors support yearly clinical research workshops to help young investigators get off to a strong start designing and running cancer clinical trials. These workshops recruit top researchers from around the world to present lectures and participate in discussions about all aspects of clinical trials, from statistical methodology to practical matters like how to build a career, get published, and maintain funding. The workshops are interactive. Junior faculty are required to come with a draft concept for a clinical trial that they have written. During the workshops, participants critique each other's proposals and advisors counsel the young investigators to improve the study designs. These workshops involve feverish work by all involved, but the young investigators leave the workshop with both a solid foundation in clinical trial principles and a clinical protocol suitable for submission to their institution. Often, it is in these studies that young investigators first take on the role of principal investigator. A collateral benefit of participation is ongoing professional connections stemming from both the meeting itself and participation in alumni groups maintained by each workshop organization.

The first of these workshops, starting in 1996, was the AACR/ASCO Educational Workshop "Methods in Clinical Cancer Research," most often referred to as the Vail Workshop based on its location in Vail, Colorado, USA [149]. In 1999, the program was replicated in Europe, with the establishment of the ECCO-AACR-EORTC-ESMO Workshop on Methods in Clinical Cancer Research, conducted in Flims, Switzerland [150]. More recently, similar workshops have started in Saudi Arabia [151] and Australia [152].

The amount of financial aid available to support participation of investigators from LMICs varies. While the Vail conference has attracted participants from LMICs, financial support is not offered. On the other hand, in the case of the most recent Saudi Arabian workshop, both travel and workshop costs were entirely absorbed by the conference organizers. The ACORD conference held in Australia offers fellowships to mitigate travel and accommodation costs and will in the event of financial hardship waive the conference fee. Similarly, the FLIMS conference allows applicants from countries with limited resources to request an exemption from the workshop participation fee.

Conclusion

In coming decades, the very success of worldwide development efforts, decreased morbidity and mortality from infectious diseases, fewer childhood and maternal deaths, an upward shift in population age with better family planning, and better food security will drive cancer and other NCDs to the center stage of global health priorities. To know which policies and interventions will succeed in addressing that coming need, cancer research directed at regions undergoing such developments needs to start now. The researchers and clinicians that will direct cancer care are already in training, perhaps benefiting from some of the opportunities described above. Training is not enough, though, as most of these skilled workers will not remain in LMICs unless the prospect exists for career-spanning research support.

The public sector, governments and international organizations included, is the largest overall funder of research and development around the world, although charitable foundations have had tremendous impact in the last decade fighting HIV/AIDS, tuberculosis, and malaria. The next generation of LMIC researchers will need to put together a patchwork of funding from these traditional donors, but be open to searching for funding from other sources such as cancer advocacy organizations, scientific and clinical professional societies, and pharmaceutical partners. In time, as development efforts take hold, LMICs themselves will need to shoulder an increasing proportion of the research agenda, as is already taking place within the BRICS.

Acknowledgments The authors wish to acknowledge the contribution of background material from the following individuals and organizations: Gail Pitts, NCI Division of Extramural Affairs; Marianne Henderson, Office of Division Operations and Analysis, NCI Division of Cancer Epidemiology and Genetics; Makeda Williams, NCI Center for Global Health; Klora Katz, Fogarty International Center, NIH; Fiona Reddington, Head of Clinical and Population Research Funding, Strategy and Research Funding, CRUK; Luis Gabriel Cuervo Amore and Elena Villanueva, PAHO; Olaf Kelm, IARC; Matias Tuler, WHO; Michael Strange, GlaxoSmithKline.

References

1. Alwan A, editor. Global status report on noncommunicable diseases 2010. Geneva: World Health Organization; 2011.
2. Irikefe V, Vaidyanathan G, Nordling L, et al. Science in Africa: the view from the front line. Nature. 2011;474:556–9.
3. Adewole I, Martin D, Willaims M, et al. Building capacity for sustainable research programmes for cancer in Africa. Nat Rev Clin Oncol. 2014;11:251–9.
4. Bloom D, Cafiero E, Jané-Llopis E, et al. The global economic burden of noncommunicable diseases. Geneva: World Economic Forum; 2011.
5. World Bank. Country and Lending Groups. http://data.worldbank.org/about/country-and-lending-groups (2014). Accessed 23 Oct 2014.
6. Rebbeck TR, editor. Handbook for cancer research in Africa. Brazzaville: World Health Organization, Regional Office for Africa; 2013.

7. Viergever RF. Aid alignment for global health research: the role of HIROs. Health Res Policy Syst. 2011;9:12.
8. International Cancer Research Partnership database. https://www.icrpartnership.org/database.cfm. Accessed 23 Oct 2014.
9. Global Oncology, Inc. Cancer resource map. http://globalonc.org/Projects/cancer-resource-map/. Accessed 23 Oct 2014.
10. Bliss K, editor. Key players in global health: how Brazil, Russia, India, China and South Africa are influencing the game. Washington, DC: Center for Strategic and International Studies; 2010.
11. Chaturvedi S, Thorsteindótir H. BRICS and South-South cooperation in medicine: emerging trends in research and entrepreneurial collaborations. RIS Discussion Papers, #177. New Delhi: Research and Information Systems for Developing Countries; 2012.
12. Conselho Nacional de Desenvolvimento Científico e Tecnológico. http://www.cnpq.br/web/guest/apresentacao13. Accessed 23 Oct 2014.
13. The World Academy of Sciences. TWAS-CNPq Postgraduate Fellowship Programme http://www.twas.org/opportunity/twas-cnpq-postgraduate-fellowship-programme. Accessed 23 Oct 2014.
14. International Development Research Center. Who can apply: IDRC International Fellowships. http://www.idrc.ca/EN/Funding/WhoCanApply/Pages/IDRC-International-Fellowships-Program.aspx. Accessed 23 Oct 2014.
15. International Development Research Center. Who can apply: IDRC research awards. http://www.idrc.ca/EN/Funding/WhoCanApply/Pages/Internships-at-IDRC.aspx. Accessed 23 Oct 2014.
16. Canadian Institute for Health Research. ResearchNet: current funding opportunities. https://www.researchnet-recherchenet.ca/rnr16/LoginServlet. Accessed 23 Oct 2014.
17. International Development Research Center. Global Health Research Initiative. http://www.idrc.ca/EN/Programs/Global_Health_Policy/Global_Health_Research_Initiative/Pages/Approach.aspx. Accessed 23 Oct 2014.
18. Department of International Cooperation, Chinese Ministry of Science and Technology. China International Science and Technology Cooperation. http://www.cistc.gov.cn/english-version/. Accessed 23 Oct 2014.
19. Department of International Cooperation, Chinese Ministry of Science and Technology. China-ASEAN Science and Technology Partnership Program. http://www.cistc.com/China-ASEAN/English/?column=831. Accessed 23 Oct 2014.
20. Department of International Cooperation, Chinese Ministry of Science and Technology. Castep Launch Ceremony. http://www.cistc.gov.cn/englishversion/FeaturesInfo.asp?column=710. Accessed 23 Oct 2014.
21. Department of International Cooperation, Chinese Ministry of Science and Technology. Talented young scientist program. http://www.cistc.com/China-ASEAN/English/info.asp?column=839&id=82350. Accessed 23 Oct 2014.
22. National Natural Science Foundation of China. http://www.nsfc.gov.cn/Portals/1/fj/pdf/01-01.pdf. Accessed 23 Oct 2014.
23. National Natural Science Foundation of China. International activities. http://www.nsfc.gov.cn/publish/portal1/tab159/info24587.htm. Accessed 23 Oct 2014.
24. National Natural Science Foundation of China. 年度自然科学基金外国青年学者研究基金项目指南. http://www.nsfc.gov.cn/publish/portal0/tab38/info39844.htm. Accessed 23 Oct 2014.
25. Bureau of International Co-operation, Chinese Academy of Sciences. CAS President's International Fellowship Initiative (PIFI).http://english.bic.cas.cn/AF/Fe/201408/t20140807_125680.html. Accessed 23 Oct 2014.
26. Chinese Scholarship Council. Introduction to Chinese Government Scholarships. http://en.csc.edu.cn/Laihua/scholarshipdetailen.aspx?cid=97&id=2070. Accessed 23 Oct 2014.

27. United National Educational, Scientific, and Cultural Organization. UNESCO/People's Republic of China (The Great Wall) Co-Sponsored Fellowships Programme. http://www. unesco.org/new/en/fellowships/programmes/unescopeoples-republic-of-china-the-great-wall-co-sponsored-fellowships-programme/. Accessed 23 Oct 2014.
28. European Commission. Participant Portal H2020 Online Manual. http://ec.europa.eu/research/participants/docs/h2020-funding-guide/index_en.htm. Accessed 23 Oct 2014.
29. European Commission. Individual Fellowships. http://ec.europa.eu/research/mariecurieactions/about-msca/actions/if/index_en.htm. Accessed 23 Oct 2014.
30. European Research Council. Statistics. http://erc.europa.eu/statistics-0. Accessed 23 Oct 2014.
31. European Research Council. Funding schemes. http://erc.europa.eu/funding-schemes. Accessed 23 Oct 2014.
32. European Research Council. Call for proposals. http://erc.europa.eu/call-proposals. Accessed 23 Oct 2014.
33. European and Developing Countries Clinical Trial Partnerships. Applying for Grants. http://www.edctp.org/calls-and-grants/applying-for-grants/. Accessed 23 Oct 2014.
34. Institut national de la santé et de la recherche médicale. From calls for proposals. http://english.inserm.fr/calls-for-proposals/. Accessed 23 Oct 2014.
35. Institut national de la santé et de la recherche médicale. List of INSERM's international cooperation agreements. http://english.inserm.fr/content/download/53454/307700/file/accords_cooperation_internationaux_va.pdf. Accessed 23 Oct 2014.
36. Institut national de la santé et de la recherche médicale. Practical information. http://english.inserm.fr/what-s-inserm/international-policy/practical-information. Accessed 23 Oct 2014.
37. Institut national de la santé et de la recherche médicale. Other sources of funding to support international collaborative research. http://english.inserm.fr/what-s-inserm/international-policy/other-sources-of-funding-to-support-international-collaborative-research. Accessed 23 Oct 2014.
38. Institut national de la santé et de la recherche médicale. Budget 2013. http://www.inserm.fr/qu-est-ce-que-l-inserm/missions-de-l-institut/budget-2014/activite-scientifique-par-thematique-de-recherche-et-par-nature-de-depenses. Accessed 23 Oct 2014.
39. Institut National du Cancer de France. L'état prévisionnel des recettes et des dépenses 2013. http://www.e-cancer.fr/linstitut-national-du-cancer/presentation/budget. Accessed 23 Oct 2014.
40. Institut National du Cancer de France. Les appels à projets et à candidatures de l'INCa. http://www.e-cancer.fr/aap. Accessed 23 Oct 2014.
41. Institut National du Cancer de France. Modalités d'organisation des appels à proje. http://www.e-cancer.fr/aap/les-procedures. Accessed 23 Oct 2014.
42. Indian Council of Medical Research. Thrust areas of research. http://icmr.nic.in/thrust/thrust.htm. Accessed 23 Oct 2014.
43. Indian Council of Medical Research. Guidelines for international collaboration/research. http://icmr.nic.in/guide.htm. Accessed 23 Oct 2014.
44. Indian Council of Medical Research. ICMR International fellowship programme for Indian biomedical scientists. http://icmr.nic.in/ifc_research.htm. Accessed 23 Oct 2014.
45. Indian Council of Medical Research. ICMR international fellowship program for biomedical scientists from developing countries. http://icmr.nic.in/ihd_research.htm. Accessed 23 Oct 2014.
46. Government of the Republic of South Africa. South African Medical Research Council Act of 1991. http://www.mrc.ac.za/about/MRCAct.pdf. Accessed 23 Oct 2014.
47. South African Medical Research Council. Scholarships and grants. http://www.mrc.ac.za/researchdevelopment/opportunity.htm. Accessed 23 Oct 2014.
48. South African Medical Research Council. Self-initiated research grants guidelines and information. http://www.mrc.ac.za/funding/university.htm. Accessed 23 Oct 2014.
49. South African Medical Research Council. SAMRC annual performance plan for FY 2014/2015. http://www.mrc.ac.za/publications/MRCAnnualPerformancePlan.pdf. Accessed 23 Oct 2014.

50. South African Medical Research Council. Local (non-MRC) and international funding. http://www.mrc.ac.za/funding/newsitems.htm#BasicCancer. Accessed 23 Oct 2014.
51. South African Medical Research Council. SAMRC strategic plan for FY2014/15–2018/19. http://www.mrc.ac.za/publications/MRCStrategicPlan.pdf. Accessed 23 Oct 2014.
52. South African Medical Research Council. Request for applications: national and international conferences. http://www.mrc.ac.za/funding/conferences.htm. Accessed 23 Oct 2014.
53. Russian Science Fund. Конкурсы. http://rscf.ru/contests. Accessed 23 Oct 2014.
54. Russian Science Fund. (Результаты заявочной кампании конкурса РНФ на финансирование проектов международных научных групп). http://www.rscf.ru/sites/default/files/stat_004.pdf. Accessed 23 Oct 2014.
55. Russian Fund for Fundamental Research. Международная деятельность РФФИ: http://www.rfbr.ru/rffi/ru/international. Accessed 23 Oct 2014.
56. Russian Fund for Fundamental Research.Финансирование: http://www.rfbr.ru/rffi/ru/funding. Accessed 23 Oct 2014.
57. Russian Fund for Fundamental Research. Отчет о деятельности Россиского фонда фундаментальных исследований в 2013 году. http://www.rfbr.ru/rffi/getimage/%D0%9E%D1%82%D1%87%D0%B5%D1%82+%D0%A0%D0%A4%D0%A4%D0%98+%D0%B7%D0%B0+2013+%D0%B3%D0%BE%D0%B4.pdf?objectId=1897742. Accessed 23 Oct 2014.
58. Russian Fund for Fundamental Research. Международные конкурсы: http://www.rfbr.ru/rffi/ru/international_contests. Accessed 23 Oct 2014.
59. Swedish International Development Agency. Research cooperation. http://www.sidaresearch.se/research-cooperation.aspx. Accessed 23 Oct 2014.
60. The Scientific and Technological Research Council of Turkey. Announcements. http://www.tubitak.gov.tr/en. Accessed 23 Oct 2014.
61. UK Medical Research Council. Browse funding opportunities. http://www.mrc.ac.uk/funding/browse/. Accessed 23 Oct 2014.
62. UK Medical Research Council. ODA IATI data CY 2013 TOTAL FV 2. http://www.mrc.ac.uk/documents/xls-csv/oda-iati-data-cy-2013-total-fv-2/. Accessed 23 Oct 2014.
63. UK Medical Research Council. Browse funding opportunities. http://www.mrc.ac.uk/funding/browse/. Accessed 23 Oct 2014
64. UK Medical Research Council. Remit and scope; http://www.mrc.ac.uk/funding/science-areas/global-health/remit-and-scope/. Accessed 23 Oct 2014.
65. Government of the United States of America. President Obama's global development policy and the global health initiative 2010. http://www.whitehouse.gov/sites/default/files/Global_Health_Fact_Sheet.pdf. Accessed 23 Oct 2014.
66. President's emergency plan for AIDS relief. http://www.pepfar.gov/. Accessed 23 Oct 2014.
67. US National Institutes of Health. Research portfolio online reporting tools (RePORT)http://report.nih.gov/. Accessed 23 Oct 2014.
68. US National Institutes of Health. Tabular data, President's budget request 2014. http://officeofbudget.od.nih.gov/pdfs/FY15/FY2015_Overview.pdf. Accessed 23 Oct 2014.
69. US National Cancer Institute. National Cancer Act of 1937. http://legislative.cancer.gov/history/1937. Accessed 23 Oct 2014.
70. US National Institutes of Health. Grants and funding. http://grants.nih.gov/grants/oer.htm. Accessed 23 Oct 2014.
71. US National Institutes of Health. Information for foreign applicants and grantees. http://grants.nih.gov/grants/foreign/index.htm. Accessed 23 Oct 2014.
72. US National Cancer Institute. NCI FY2012 Fact book. http://obf.cancer.gov/financial/attachments/12Factbk.pdf. Accessed 23 Oct 2014.
73. US National Institutes of Health. Types of grant programs. http://grants.nih.gov/grants/funding/funding_program.htm. Accessed 23 Oct 2014.
74. US National Cancer Institute. 2013 Division of extramural affairs annual report. 2014
75. Trimble EL, Abrams JS, Meyer RM, et al. Improving cancer outcomes through international collaboration in academic center treatment trials. J Clin Oncol. 2009;27:5109–14.

76. US National Cancer Institute, Clinical Therapy Evaluation Program. Active Agreements 2014. http://ctep.cancer.gov/protocolDevelopment/docs/ctep_active_agreements.xlsx. Accessed 23 Oct 2014.
77. US National Cancer Institute, Clinical Therapy Evaluation Program. Letter of Intent. http://ctep.cancer.gov/protocolDevelopment/letter_of_intent.htm. Accessed 23 Oct 2014.
78. US National Cancer Institute, Office of HIV and AIDS Malignancy. Research on malignancies in the context of HIV/AIDS. http://oham.cancer.gov/funding/. Accessed 23 Oct 2014.
79. AIDS Malignancy Consortium. http://pub.emmes.com/study/amc/public/index.htm. Accessed 23 Oct 2014.
80. US National Cancer Institute, Center for Global Health. CGH Short Term Scientist Exchange Program (STSEP). http://www.cancer.gov/aboutnci/organization/global-health/funding-and-training/scientist-exchange. Accessed 23 Oct 2014.
81. US National Institutes of Health. RFA-CA-13-015. http://grants.nih.gov/grants/guide/rfa-files/RFA-CA-13-015.html. Accessed 23 Oct 2014.
82. US National Institutes of Health. NOT-CA-14-055. http://grants.nih.gov/grants/guide/notice-files/NOT-CA-14-055.html. Accessed 23 Oct 2014.
83. US National Cancer Institute. Cancer Prevention Fellowship Program. http://cpfp.nci.nih.gov/curriculum/index.shtml. Accessed 23 Oct 2014.
84. US National Cancer Institute, Center for Global Health. Trans-NIH Regional Grant Writing & Scientific Peer Review Workshops. http://www.cancer.gov/aboutnci/organization/global-health/research-programs-initiatives/trans-nih-regional-workshops. Accessed 23 Oct 2014.
85. US National Institutes of Health, Fogarty International Center. Congressional Justification for Fiscal Year 2014. http://www.fic.nih.gov/About/Budget/Pages/2014.aspx#appropriation. Accessed 23 Oct 2014.
86. De Martel C, Ferlay J, Franceschi F. Global burden of cancers attributable to infections in 2008: a review and synthetic analysis. Lancet Oncol. 2012;13:607–15.
87. US Human Genome Research Institute. Ethical, Legal, and Social Implications (ELSI) funding opportunities. http://www.genome.gov/10000930. Accessed 23 Oct 2014.
88. US National Cancer Institute. Funding opportunities by type. http://www.cancer.gov/researchandfunding/funding/announcements. Accessed 23 Oct 2014.
89. US National Institute of Allergy and Infectious Diseases. Opportunities and announcements. http://www.niaid.nih.gov/researchfunding/ann/pages/default.aspx. Accessed 23 Oct 2014.
90. US National Heart, Lung and Blood Institute. NHLBI Grants and Contracts: Funding Opportunity Announcements (FOAs).https://www.nhlbi.nih.gov/research/funding/opportunities/. Accessed 23 Oct 2014.
91. US National Institutes of Diabetes and Digestive and Kidney Diseases. Current funding opportunities. http://www.niddk.nih.gov/research-funding/current-opportunities/Pages/FO.aspx.
92. US National Human Genome Research Institute. NHGRI Funding Opportunity: Research. http://www.genome.gov/10000991. Accessed 23 Oct 2014.
93. US National Institutes of Health. Funding opportunities and notices. http://grants.nih.gov/grants/guide/index.html. Accessed 23 Oct 2014.
94. United States Agency for International Development. Partnerships for Enhanced Engagement in Research (PEER). http://www.usaid.gov/what-we-do/science-technolog-and-innovation/international-research-science-programs/partnerships. Accessed 23 Oct 2014.
95. US National Academy of Sciences Partnerships for Enhanced Engagement in Research (PEER). http://sites.nationalacademies.org/PGA/PEER/PGA_147214. Accessed 23 Oct 2014.
96. United States Agency for International Development. Country Strategies (CDCS). http://www.usaid.gov/results-and-data/planning/country-strategies-cdcs.
97. United States Agency for International Development. US Global Development Lab. https://www.grantinterface.com/Common/LogOn.aspx?eqs=wG-r-jJPukYm24Q4inQrFQ2. Accessed 23 Oct 2014.
98. Institut Pasteur. All the calls for applications. http://www.pasteur.fr/en/international/institut-pasteur-around-world/calls-proposals/all-calls-applications. Accessed 23 Oct 2014.

99. Institut Pasteur. Courses 2014. http://www.pasteur.fr/en/international/international-network-courses/international-courses/all-institut-pasteur-international-network-courses/courses-2014. Accessed 23 Oct 2014.
100. World Bank. Scholarships. http://wbi.worldbank.org/wbi/scholarships. Accessed 23 Oct 2014.
101. Islamic Development Bank. Shttp://www.isdb.org/. Accessed 23 Oct 2014.
102. The World Academy of Sciences. TWAS annual report 2013. http://www.twas.org/sites/default/files/twas_an_rep_13_web.pdf. Accessed 23 Oct 2014.
103. The World Academy of Sciences. Opportunities. http://www.twas.org/opportunities. Accessed 23 Oct 2014.
104. Union for International Cancer Control. Fellowships. http://www.uicc.org/programmes/global-education-and-training-initiative-geti/fellowships. Accessed 23 Oct 2014.
105. World Health Organization. Research for universal health coverage: World health report 2013. Geneva: World Health Organization; 2013.
106. World Health Organization. The WHO Strategy on research for health. Geneva: World Health Organization; 2012.
107. International Agency for Research on Cancer. Facts and Figures. http://training.iarc.fr/en/about/facts_figures.php. Accessed 23 Oct 2014.
108. International Agency for Research on Cancer. Education and Training. http://training.iarc.fr/en/fellowships/postdoc.php. Accessed 23 Oct 2014.
109. International Agency for Research on Cancer. Summer School in Lyon. http://training.iarc.fr/en/courses/summerschool/index.php. Accessed 23 Oct 2014.
110. WHO Special Programme for Research and Training in Tropical Diseases. Grants and other funding activities. http://www.who.int/tdr/grants/en/. Accessed 23 Oct 2014.
111. World Health Organization. WHO regional offices. http://www.who.int/about/regions/en/. Accessed 23 Oct 2014.
112. Pan American Health Organization. Resolution CD49.R10: Policy on Research for Health, 2009. http://new.paho.org/hq/dmdocuments/2009/CD49-R10-Eng.pdf. Accessed 23 Oct 2014.
113. Villanueva EC, de Abreu DR, Cuervo LG, et al. HRweb Americas: a tool to facilitate better research governance in Latin America and the Caribbean. Cad Saude Publica. 2012;28:2003–8.
114. Centro Internacionla de Entrenamiento e Investigaciones Médicas. http://www.cideim.org.co/cideim/. Accessed 23 Oct 2014.
115. Alger J, Gomez L, Jaramillo A, et al. Meeting of the inter-regional network of reference centers for effective training in planning and evaluation courses on health research projects, April 2010. Rev Med Hondur. 2010;78:96–9.
116. Organization of American States. OAS and PAHO to Offer Scholarships to Promote Health and Research Issues in the Americas. http://www.oas.org/en/media_center/press_release.asp?sCodigo=E-047/14. Accessed 23 Oct 2015.
117. Organization of American States. Call for applications for PAHO-OAS health scholarships in Brazil. http://www.paho.org/hq/index.php?option=com_content&view=article&id=9697:call-for-applications-for-paho-oas-health-scholarships-in-brazil&Itemid=2&lang=en. Accessed 23 Oct 2014.
118. Bill and Melinda Gates Foundation. Grant Opportunities. http://www.gatesfoundation.org/How-We-Work/General-Information/Grant-Opportunities. Accessed 23 Oct 2014.
119. Bill and Melinda Gates Foundation. Grand Challenges Grant Opportunities. http://gcgh.grandchallenges.org/GrantOpportunities/Pages/default.aspx. Accessed 23 Oct 2014.
120. Bill and Melinda Gates Foundation. Open Concept Memo Global Health Grants. http://www.gatesfoundation.org/How-We-Work/General-Information/Grant-Opportunities/Open-Concept-Memo-Global-Health-Grants. Accessed 23 Oct 2014.
121. Cancer Research UK. 2013/14 Annual Report. http://www.cancerresearchuk.org/sites/default/files/annual_report_and_accounts_2013-14.pdf. Accessed 23 Oct 2014.
122. Cancer Research UK. Applying for Funding. http://www.cancerresearchuk.org/funding-for-researchers/applying-for-funding. Accessed 23 Oct 2014.

123. The Global Fund to Fight AIDS, Tuberculosis and Malaria. Funding and spending. http://www.theglobalfund.org/en/about/fundingspending/. Accessed 23 Oct 2014.
124. The Global Fund to Fight AIDS, Tuberculosis and Malaria. Grant Portfolio. http://portfolio.theglobalfund.org/. Accessed 23 Oct 2014.
125. Susan G. Komen Foundation. Funding Opportunities. http://ww5.komen.org/GrantsCentral/InternationalGrants/FundingOpportunities/FundingOpportunities.html. Accessed 23 Oct 2014.
126. Susan G. Komen Foundation. Consolidated Financial Statement and Supplementary Information. http://ww5.komen.org/uploadedFiles/Content/AboutUs/Financial/Susan%20G%20Komen%20Financial%20Statements%20FY13.pdf. Accessed 23 Oct 2014.
127. Susan G. Komen Foundation. Current Funding Opportunities. http://ww5.komen.org/ResearchGrants/FundingOpportunities.html. Accessed 23 Oct 2014.
128. Susan G. Komen Foundation. Research World Map. http://ww5.komen.org/ResearchWorldMap.aspx. Accessed 23 Oct 2014.
129. Wellcome Trust. Current grant portfolio and 2012/13 grant funding data. http://www.wellcome.ac.uk/stellent/groups/corporatesite/@msh_publishing_group/documents/web_document/wts058353.pdf. Accessed 23 Oct 2014.
130. Wellcome Trust. Strategic Plan 2010-20 Extraordinary Opportunities. http://www.wellcome.ac.uk/stellent/groups/corporatesite/@policy_communications/documents/web_document/WTDV027438.pdf. Accessed 23 Oct 2014.
131. Wellcome Trust. Public health and tropical medicine. http://www.wellcome.ac.uk/Funding/Biomedical-science/Funding-schemes/Fellowships/Public-health-and-tropical-medicine/index.htm. Accessed 23 Oct 2014.
132. Wellcome Trust. International. http://www.wellcome.ac.uk/Funding/index.htm. Accessed 19 October 2015.
133. Wellcome Trust. Major Overseas Programs. http://www.wellcome.ac.uk/Funding/International/Major-Overseas-Programmes/index.htm. Accessed 23 Oct 2014.
134. Wellcome Trust. Fellowship Schemes. http://www.wellcomedbt.org/fellowships.html. Accessed 23 Oct 2014.
135. World Cancer Research Fund. Apply for a research grant. http://www.wcrf.org/apply. Accessed 23 Oct 2014.
136. GlaxoSmithKline, plc. Trust in Science LATAM. http://www.gsk.com/en-gb/research/research-funding/trust-in-science-latam/. Accessed 23 Oct 2014.
137. GlaxoSmithKline, plc. Trust in Science Africa. http://www.gsk.com/en-gb/research/research-funding/trust-in-science-africa/. Accessed 23 Oct 2014
138. GlaxoSmithKline, plc. GSK announces new strategic investments in Africa to increase access to medicines, build capacity and deliver sustainable growth. http://www.developingcountriesunit.gsk.com/Our-Stories/News/GSK-announces-new-strategic-investments-in-Africa-to-increase-access-to-medicines-build-capacity-and-deliver-sustainable_. Accessed 23 Oct 2014.
139. American Association for Cancer Research. Funding Opportunities. http://www.aacr.org/funding/Pages/funding-listing.aspx. Accessed 23 Oct 2014.
140. Litchman SM. Global initiatives to enhance cancer care in areas of limited resources: what ASCO members are doing and how you can become involved. Am Soc Clin Oncol Educ Book. 411-413; 2013.
141. Conquer Cancer Foundation. International Development and Education Award. http://www.conquercancerfoundation.org/cancer-professionals/funding-opportunities/international-development-and-education-award. Accessed 23 Oct 2014.
142. Conquer Cancer Foundation International Innovation Grant. http://www.conquercancerfoundation.org/cancer-professionals/funding-opportunities/international-innovation-grant. Accessed 23 Oct 2014.
143. American Society for Clinical Oncology. International Clinical Trials Workshops. http://www.asco.org/international-programs/international-clinical-trials-workshops. Accessed 23 Oct 2014.

144. Conquer Cancer Foundation. Long-term international fellowships. http://www.conquercancerfoundation.org/long-term-international-fellowship. Accessed 23 Oct 2014.
145. Conquer Cancer Foundation. Cancer Research Map. http://www.conquercancerfoundation.org/cancer-professionals/grants-awards/cancer-research-map. Accessed 23 Oct 2014.
146. Conquer Cancer Foundation Complete listing of funding opportunities. http://www.conquercancerfoundation.org/cancer-professionals/funding-opportunities/complete-listing-of-funding-opportunities. Accessed 23 Oct 2014.
147. European Society for Medical Oncology ESMO Fellowship Offers. http://www.esmo.org/Career-Development/Oncology-Fellowships/Fellowship-Offers. Accessed 23 Oct 2014.
148. European Society for Medical Oncology. External Oncology Fellowship Opportunities. http://www.esmo.org/Career-Development/Oncology-Fellowships/External-Fellowships. Accessed 23 Oct 2014.
149. American Association for Cancer Research. General information. http://vailworkshop.org/Pages/GeneralInformation.aspx. Accessed 23 Oct 2014.
150. European Cancer Organisation. Clinical trials workshop (Flims). http://www.ecco-org.eu/Education/Clinical-trials-workshop. Accessed 23 Oct 2014.
151. King Abdulaziz City for Science and Technology. Call for applications. http://mcrw.kacst.edu.sa/. Accessed 23 Oct 2014.
152. Australia & Asia Pacific Clinical Oncology Research Development. http://acord.org.au/. Accessed 23 Oct 2014.

Chapter 9
International Collaboration in Cancer Research

Daniela Cristina Stefan and Eduardo Seleiro

Abstract International research collaboration, facilitated by the progress of communication and travel, stimulates the scientific progress by combining the strengths of the partnering institutions.

For developing countries, with limited capacity to control a relatively high burden of disease, associating with institutions from resource-rich countries to undertake research is an efficient way of finding solutions to local health issues, with the added benefit of building up research capacity. Such collaborations should reside on sound principles—as illustrated in this chapter—if they are to benefit all partners. Powerful international organizations like the International Agency for Research on Cancer and the National Cancer Institute are conducting large international studies, with the participation of many limited-resource partners.

Keywords International collaboration • Cancer research • International Agency for Research on Cancer • National Cancer Institute

In today's increasingly interconnected and interdependent community of nations, international collaboration in research is increasingly becoming the norm. Exploiting the synergies of multinational research groups has the potential to persuade funding agencies, to enhance the scientific (and practical) value of the studies, and to facilitate skill transfers. Sometimes the required power of a study cannot be achieved without involving several research units, which may be located in different countries, each contributing a number of cases. At other times, containing globally spreading infectious agents like HIV or, more recently, the Ebola virus, requires the combined efforts of scientists from various countries.

D.C. Stefan, M.D., Ph.D. (✉)
South African Medical Research Council, Francie van Zyl, Parrow, Cape Town, South Africa
e-mail: Cristina.Stefan@mrc.ac.za

E. Seleiro, Ph.D.
International Agency for Research on Cancer, 150 Cours Albert Thomas, Lyon, France
e-mail: selerioe@iarc.fr

© Springer International Publishing Switzerland 2016
D.C. Stefan (ed.), *Cancer Research and Clinical Trials in Developing Countries*, DOI 10.1007/978-3-319-18443-2_9

International collaboration in research is even more necessary for developing nations, where a relatively high burden of disease is often poorly controlled, because it is insufficiently researched. The situation was summarized by the Global Forum for Health Research in the "10/90 gap" concept, which states that only 10 % of the world research and development money is spent on highly prevalent diseases which affect 90 % of the population [1]. By partnering with resource-rich countries in undertaking research on regional health challenges, developing countries obtain easier access to funding, can draw on the capacity of experienced scientists to conduct studies, can obtain training for various skills related to research, and can access sophisticated laboratory facilities. Also, a portion of the funds can be directed towards infrastructure development and the supplementation of scientists' salaries.

As most of the countries with high resources are situated in the northern hemisphere, the cooperation in research with lower-income countries is known as North–South cooperation. Presently, some of the middle-income countries in the South have managed to develop their research capacity and experience to the level where they can actually mentor other Southern countries while working side-by-side at common research, forming South–South collaborations [2]. The main obstacle in the way of growing South–South common research initiatives is the difficulty in obtaining funding.

The essential condition for success in a North–South partnership is fairness. This enterprise is, at its inception, far from a partnership of equals. The funding is almost always provided by Northern agencies, and the expertise and facilities balance is skewed towards the North. Moreover, the Northern partner is regarded by the funders as carrying more responsibility for correct budget spending and for the good scientific quality of the output.

Examples are described in the literature of collaborations that did not best serve the interest of the developing country involved. In numerous cases, the southern partner was simply a donor of samples which were processed in the North, without any further participation. Papers are known to have been published without acknowledging the developing country contribution [3]. In some cases where a northern scientist was seconded to the research site in the South, a major portion of the budget was simply used to cover the salary and expenses of that expert [4]. Another important issue may be the choice of research theme. The findings of the studies should serve to answer major health problems in the South rather than issues only relevant to the northern partner.

A few valuable lessons were learnt along the way from the practice of international research partnerships. One of them is that all collaborators should participate from the onset in planning and budgeting the studies. The research questions, approved by all sides, should be relevant to all. Critical research instruments such as questionnaires and informed consent forms need to be written in collaboration with the scientists from the country where the research will take place, in the language of the research subjects. Avoiding unilateral publication of papers by one of the sides in the partnership requires a publishing plan, drawn right from the beginning of the collaboration, stipulating the authors and their roles [5]. New papers may be proposed along the way according to a pre-agreed protocol.

Divergent opinions sometimes arise around which ethical review committees should approve the studies. Unilateral approval in the North was at times denounced as an attempt to impose certain moral values on the South, coupled with distrust in the capacity of their ethical review system. But submission to ethical scrutiny in the North is often a condition for releasing the funds. On the other hand, approval by local ethical structures in the South offers a guarantee that the research capacity engaged is adequate, that the informed consent will be obtained in an appropriate manner, and that the study will be conducted in accordance with the communities' expectations. It is therefore clear that ethical approval in all participating institutions is required to start the research [6].

To ensure that the collaboration will contribute to increasing the research capacity according to the needs of partners, the budget should clearly specify the objectives (infrastructure and skills), how will they be achieved, including a timeframe, and how much will be spent on each objective. A number of Masters and PhD fellowships should be agreed upon during the planning period and provisions for postdoctoral career prospects should be made. For low- and middle-income countries (LMICs), the brain drain is a persistent threat, and the best approach to minimizing it includes postdoctoral fellowships which ensure adequate remuneration, often as a top-up to salary, in the context of a meaningful research program. Such fellowships should also provide opportunities for scientists from southern countries to visit northern institutions, to forge new professional connections and maintain old ones (personal relationships have proven to be very important in the viability of the cooperation), and to maintain their knowledge and skills at the highest level. This is best done when the North–South collaboration is a long-term one, perhaps for a decade or longer [7].

The Swiss Commission for Research Partnerships with Developing Countries (SCRPDC), a Platform of the Swiss Academy of Science, issued a publication in 2012 which integrates their experience obtained in international research collaboration. The second edition appeared in 2014 and contains 11 principles whose application should result in an equitable and rewarding partnership for all organizations involved [8]. These principles are summarized in Table 9.1.

Among the numerous organizations and international institutions that promote international research cooperation, the World Health Organization's International Agency for Research on Cancer (IARC) is one of the most prominent. The following section details the activities of the IARC.

The International Agency for Research on Cancer

Collaboration is at the heart of the mission and activities of the IARC, which was created in 1965 as an autonomous specialized agency of the WHO specifically dedicated to promoting collaboration in cancer research. The role of IARC as a catalyst for international collaboration is highlighted in Article 1 of its Statute:

The objective of the International Agency for Research on Cancer shall be to promote international collaboration in cancer research. […]

Table 9.1 Principles for successful international research collaboration, according to SCRPDC

Principle	Comment
Set the agenda together	The research questions and the modalities of solving them should be agreed from the onset. Rules governing the contribution of partners in the process should be spelled out
Interact with stakeholders	Who are the beneficiaries of the research findings (e.g., governmental departments)? They should be consulted when formulating the research questions, and sometimes along the way, to ensure maximum relevance for the society
Clarify responsibilities	Establish who does what, considering also skills, experience, and preferences. This should be part of a Memorandum of Understanding
Account to beneficiaries	Report to funders, but also observe the accountability to science in general and society, or a specific group of it (e.g., patients whose disease is being researched). Establish how reporting will be done
Promote mutual learning	Put adequate structures in place to facilitate meetings where scientists can exchange experience, ideas, opinions, and plans related to common research
Enhance capacities	While southern partners benefit from the knowledge, technology, and know-how of the North, the latter will also use the collaboration to enhance the skills of junior scientists and to develop approaches to global health problems
Share data and networks	Information exchange is essential in a partnership. How much of it can be shared without losing potential benefits? Partners should negotiate what would be shared and how it will be used
Disseminate results	Careful selection of dissemination channels (meetings, journals, mass media) in order to reach the audience that will benefit from the research
Pool profits and merits	Authorship, copyrights, and patent rights should be decided early in the process. A system of arbitration should be agreed upon
Apply results	If the research has immediate practical consequences, users should be contacted early and be kept informed of the progress and of the results, which should be presented in an easy-to-understand format.
Secure outcomes	Infrastructure created should serve for new projects. Similarly, scientists and other personnel need to be integrated in a continued research flow once the initial project is finished

Over the past 50 years, the IARC has established itself as the hub of a worldwide network for cancer research, providing a unique environment for international exchange and cooperation. In particular, IARC has a longstanding commitment to establishing partnerships and collaborations with researchers and institutions in LMICs, supporting the development of local capacity for cancer research and cancer control.

An essential feature of IARC's approach has been the coordination of many international, multicenter collaborative research projects on cancer epidemiology. Many of these studies have been stimulated by striking observations on geographic variations in cancer patterns among different populations. Research on cancer etiology often requires large, transnational studies, particularly in the study of rarer cancers or cancers affecting specific sections of the population, such as the study of cancer patterns among disadvantaged populations in high-income countries.

Another significant approach consists of the establishment of large-scale collaborative research platforms, bringing together population-based studies with rich datasets on exposure variables and associated biological specimens. IARC has coordinated the creation of several of these research consortia, which have established unique cohorts and served as the basis for large studies in diverse parts of the world.

IARC's status as an international organization, part of WHO, and the broader UN family, its reputation for rigorous, objective, and independent research, and its well-established expertise in the coordination of international collaborative research projects facilitate the collection and sharing of both data and biospecimens between the networks of collaborating centers. IARC also has the capacity to act as a custodian of biospecimen collections for collaborating centers where conditions for long-term sample storage are challenging. The Agency also plays a leading role in the collation and evaluation of scientific information and provision of global resources on the occurrence, causes, and prevention of cancer for the research community and for policy development.

IARC has established many successful collaborations which have made major contributions to different areas of cancer research. The following paragraphs provide examples of current IARC projects, which exemplify the Agency's central role in the coordination of large-scale collaborative projects in different domains.

The Global Initiative for Cancer Registry Development

An example of IARC's role in supporting the development of collaborative networks and the development of infrastructure for cancer research is the Global Initiative for Cancer Registry Development (GICR).[1] The GICR is a multi-partner initiative coordinated by IARC to improve the availability and quality of cancer data, particularly in LMICs, by supporting improvements in the development and coverage of population-based cancer registries. The GICR approach consists of the establishment of IARC regional hubs for cancer registration, offering training and technical support to existing registries in their regions and providing assistance to enhance networking and research capacity, as well as supporting advocacy to countries for the establishment of population-based cancer registries.

Since its creation in 2011, four regional hubs have been established (in Africa, Asia, and Latin America) and two additional hubs are planned to start operations in 2015 (in the Caribbean and the Pacific Islands). The goal of the project is to produce measurable improvements in the coverage, quality, and national networking capacity of population-based cancer registries in 50 LMICs by 2018.

---

[1] For more information on this project see http://gicr.iarc.fr/

The ESTAMPA Study

The *Multicenter study of cervical cancer screening and triage with human papilloma virus testing* (ESTAMPA) aims to evaluate the feasibility of different approaches for implementation of organized HPV-based screening programs. HPV-based screening requires triage of HPV-positive women to identify true cancer precursors. The study will evaluate different triage methods (including visual inspection with acetic acid, cytology, and novel molecular techniques) to determine which method better identifies women who are most likely to have or to develop persistent HPV infection leading to high-grade cervical lesions requiring treatment.

The ESTAMPA study will recruit more than 50,000 women aged 30–64 years old in ten countries in Latin America. It will create a network of collaborating centers sharing samples and data and provide training and quality assurance for local cervical cancer screening programmes. Additionally, the study will create a biobank that will provide further opportunities for future research collaborations.

The BCNet Project

The Biobank and Cohort Building Network (BCNet) aims to provide a platform to support the development of population cohorts and biobanking facilities in LMIC.[2] The main objectives of BCNet are to promote collaboration, facilitate sharing of samples and resources among members, and the development of joint research projects. The BCNet will assist its members by developing standard protocols and guidelines for biological sample collection, storage, management, and distribution in LMICs; organize training programs and develop capacity for biobanking; search for opportunities for funding for research and training; and promote biobanking to the community and decision makers.

The BCNet project was launched in September 2013 and currently includes members from over 23 biobanks representing 14 LMICs from all the WHO regions, together with a number of national and international partner institutions from developed countries committed to collaborating in the development of biobanking in LMICs. This project provides an excellent example of where IARC can ensure the appropriate translation and adaptation of best practice in high-income countries to approaches feasible in resource-limited environments.

IARC Monographs and Handbooks of Cancer Prevention

IARC produces a number of authoritative evaluations of evidence, for example within its Monographs program and Handbooks series. In both cases, IARC is able to assemble the world's leading experts, under its auspices, to sift the available

---

[2] For more information on this project see http://bcnet.iarc.fr/about/index.php

evidence and arrive at a consensus as to whether an agent causes cancer or an intervention reduces risk of disease. All this is done with careful attention to freedom from conflict of interest. The reputation of the Agency for the quality of its research and its independence is vital to attract the experts to spend their time in this production of "public goods," which is a service to public health worldwide.

Education and Training Programme

Another dimension of IARC's research and collaboration networks is the role they play in building cancer research capacity, particularly in countries and regions where it is less developed. Education and training is one of the statutory core activities of the Agency, and since its inception IARC has had an active program of courses and fellowships integrated into its research activities. Scientists from all over the world have benefited from the training opportunities provided by IARC either in Lyon or at the sites of research projects. Moreover, collaboration with IARC offers an entry-point into a global research network, promoting access to high-quality collaborations for scientists from different backgrounds, often resulting in training exchanges and transfer of knowledge to less-developed regions. Indeed much of the training actually comes "on-the-job" from collaborations within joint projects where national researchers work alongside IARC and take responsibility for the work performed in their own population.

Finally, international collaboration for IARC also has a broader dimension that extends beyond research and capacity development to include strategic partnerships with a number of national and international organizations, ensuring the use of the Agency's work for the development of evidence-based policies and priority setting. IARC has established partnerships with numerous networks of cancer and public health professionals and with national cancer institutes and regional cancer networks, such as the *Red de Institutos Nacionales de Cáncer* in Latin America and the Asian National Cancer Centers Alliance, as well as a number of national and international non-governmental organizations, including the Union for International Cancer Control (UICC), the International Association of National Public Health Institutes (IANPHI), and the International Cancer Control Partnership (ICCP) among others. The close relationship with WHO provides a privileged channel for the translation of the scientific evidence produced by the Agency into implementable policies and guidelines, as well as access to networks of national public health and government officials through the WHO Regional Offices. More broadly, IARC collaborates with other UN agencies in the coordination of several global joint programs for cancer prevention and control in the context of the growing mobilization across the UN system on non-communicable diseases.

The importance of international collaboration and coordination, both in research and public health, is increasingly acknowledged, as demonstrated by the proliferation of new global health departments and programs in numerous institutions. IARC's extensive network of partners, built on its unique status and reputation for independence and generosity, is widely recognized as one of its major assets. IARC will continue to show leadership in international collaboration in cancer research by building on its unique experience and partnerships to address the growing need for objective, independent evidence to support the development of effective public health programs addressing the challenges posed by the rising burden of cancer worldwide.

Another prominent research organization which promotes international collaboration and has already contributed on a large scale to the development of research capacity in LMICs is the National Cancer Institute (NCI).

The National Cancer Institute

Founded in 1937 as one of the agencies (presently 11 in number) which together form the Department of Health and Human Services in USA, the NCI coordinates and funds cancer research in the country. It also develops growing international cooperation via its Centre for Global Health (CGH). Such cooperation is directed towards increasing cancer research capacity and activities in LMICs. NCI promotes cancer control planning, contributes to increasing research capacity in the partner countries, and coordinates research projects while also supporting research networks, in Latin America, China, and other regions of the world. NCI is one of the major funders of cancer research projects in USA and worldwide.

In Latin America, NCI maintains the United States-Latin America Cancer Research Network (US-LA CRN), which involves collaboration with the governments of Argentina, Brazil, Chile, Colombia, Mexico, Peru, Puerto Rico, and Uruguay to promote cancer research. US-LA CRN is currently undertaking a study on molecular profiling of breast cancer in stages II and III across participating nations [9].

The United States–China Program for Biomedical Research Cooperation has funded 109 joint projects since its inception, including numerous studies in the field of cancer research [10].

These examples illustrate the fact that international collaboration in cancer research is presently taking place on a large scale, with the support of powerful organizations such as WHO and NCI. It is important for research entities from LMICs to integrate with this trend, which has the potential to strengthen their capacity and make it easier to obtain funding for new projects. The sound principles synthesized by the SCRPDC could be used as guidance when setting up international collaborative projects.

References

1. Lewis R. Fighting the 10/90 gap. The Scientist Magazin0065, 13 May 2002. http://www.the-scientist.com/?articles.view/articleNo/14016/title/Fighting-the-10-90-Gap/. Accessed 10 Apr 2015.
2. Boshoff N. South–south research collaboration of countries in the Southern African Development Community (SADC). Scientometrics. 2010;84:481–503.

3. Rakowski C. The ugly scholar. Neocolonialism and ethical issues in international research. Am Sociol. 1993;24:69–86.
4. Costello A, Zumla A. Moving to research partnerships in developing countries. BMJ. 2000;321(7264):827–9.
5. Jentsch B, Pilley C. Research relationships between the south and the north: Cinderella and the ugly sisters? Soc Sci Med. 2003;57(10):1957–67.
6. Ravinetto R, Buvé A, Halidou T, et al. Double ethical review of North–South collaborative research: hidden paternalism or real partnership? Trop Med Int Health. 2011;6(4):527–30.
7. Chandiwana S, Ornbjerg N. Review of north–south and south–south cooperation and conditions necessary to sustain research capability in developing countries. J Health Popul Nutr. 2003;21(3):288–97.
8. Stöckli B, Wiesmann U, Lys J-A. A guide for transboundary research partnerships: 11 Principles. 2nd ed. Bern: Swiss Commission for Research Partnerships with Developing Countries (KFPE); 2012.
9. National Cancer Institute: United States-Latin America Cancer research Network (US-LA CRN). http://www.cancer.gov/aboutnci/organization/global-health/research-programs-initiatives/us-la-crn Accessed 10 Apr 2015.
10. National Cancer Institute: United States–China program for biomedical research cooperation. http://www.cancer.gov/aboutnci/organization/global-health/research-programs-initiatives/us-china-program-for-biomedical-research-cooperation Accessed 10 Apr 2015.

Chapter 10
Publication and Dissemination of Research Findings

Rebecca Johnson and David Kerr

Abstract The publishing of academic research is often the long awaited culmination of significant work by the authors. During the submission process, the author has many options that need to be considered: Which journal? Which media—print or exclusively online? Should the reader or the author pay for access, or should it be published within the emerging market of open access?

The act of publishing is necessary for several reasons; firstly, the process is peer-reviewed, which sets a quality control bench-mark that all published research has to achieve. Secondly, the access of research to a wider audience allows novel information to be accessible, which can in turn influence further research and ultimately direct treatment options.

Research that does not influence medical practice is purely an academic exercise. The gold standard of research is to direct local and national evidence-based guidelines. To facilitate this process, access to results needs to be possible at local, regional, and national levels and if possible, in real time. Furthermore, such results should be clear, concise, and focused, which permits streamline and efficient research efforts. However, further thought needs to be taken regarding factors such as intellectual property and ownership of results, of particular importance when the financial burden of research efforts is considered.

Developing nations face further issues, over and above those faced by their industrialized counterparts. Such countries tend to be resource poor, which necessitates the most efficient of treatment options. More complexity is added as these countries often face different disease burdens and pathologies, patient demographics, poorer infrastructure, and significantly reduced availability of resources.

Ultimately, up-to-date research can benefit all patients, in both developing and industrialized nations, and should be considered a necessary sphere of medicine.

R. Johnson, B.Sc., M.B.Ch.B., Ph.D. (✉)
Oxford University Hospitals NHS Trust, John Radcliffe Hospital, Oxford, Oxfordshire, UK
e-mail: Rebecca.Johnson@ouh.nhs.uk

D. Kerr, M.D., D.Sc., F.R.C.P., F.Med.Sci.
Radcliffe Department of Medicine, University of Oxford, John Radcliffe Hospital,
Oxford, Oxfordshire, UK
e-mail: david.kerr@ndcls.ox.ac.uk

© Springer International Publishing Switzerland 2016
D.C. Stefan (ed.), *Cancer Research and Clinical Trials
in Developing Countries*, DOI 10.1007/978-3-319-18443-2_10

Keywords Publication • Open access publishing • Oncology journals

Introduction

Recently, the Nobel Prize-winning physicist Peter Higgs made an astonishing announcement. "Today I wouldn't get an academic job," he told one of the UK's leading newspapers, *The Guardian*. "It's as simple as that. I don't think I would be regarded as productive enough." [1]

Higgs, who discovered one of the Universe's elementary particles, noted that quantity, not quality, is the metric by which success in the sciences is measured. Unlike in 1964, when he began his career in academia, he felt that scientists are now pressured to churn out as many papers as possible in order to retain their jobs. Had he not been nominated for the Nobel, Higgs says, he may have been fired. His scientific discovery was made possible by his era's relatively lax publishing norms, which left him time to think, dream and, above all, discover.

There is no doubt that in-depth, clearly written scholarly research has its own value: It can reshape understanding, inform policy and, for cancer research, save lives—assuming the work is accessible and implementable. However, the concept of "publish or perish" is becoming ever more firmly entrenched in academic medical careers. Promotion and career advancement depend on publication, but for readers at an early stage in establishing themselves as researchers, quality will always trump quantity. The dominant reasons for editors rejecting a peer are as follow:

- Unimportant issue studied
- Unoriginal work
- Research poorly done
- Analysis poorly done
- Conclusions not supported by results
- Poorly written/presented
- Submission does not comply with Instructions to authors

Academic publishing describes a system that is necessary in order for academic scholars to peer review the work and make it available for a wider audience. The system varies widely by field and is also always changing. Most academic work is published in journal article or book form. There is also a large body of research that exists in either a thesis or dissertation form usually found in university or college databases.

Most established academic fields have their own scientific journals and other outlets for publication though some academic journals are interdisciplinary and publish work from several distinct fields or subfields.

"There seems to be no study too fragmented, no hypothesis too trivial, no literature citation too biased or egotistical, no design too warped, no methodology too bungled, no presentation of results too inaccurate, too obscure, and too contradictory, no analysis too self-serving, no argument too circular, no conclusions too trifling or too unjustified, and no grammar and syntax too offensive for a paper to end up in print" [2].

Publication: Where and by Whom?

Having completed the research project to the highest possible standard and prepared it for publication, there are still several issues to consider.

It should be obvious who has contributed to the research and writing the paper, but the majority of medical and scientific journals will also ask each author to specify their individual contributions against a set of standard criteria—who was the idea originator; who generated samples or recruited patients; who made measurements; who collected data; who analyzed them; who produced figures, and who contributed what to writing the paper?

Some fields use ordering of the author list to indicate each person's role in a paper. The senior author in charge of the project is typically listed last. The junior author who did most of the work is typically listed first, and other contributors listed in between. There are over 200 journals that publish oncology-related research, posing the problem of where the paper should be submitted. Practice-changing research or fundamental observations which substantially challenge accepted dogma may have a chance of being accepted in world-leading general journals such as *Nature, Science, Cell, Lancet,* and *New England Journal of Medicine*, which sit at the pinnacle of medical and science literature.

A list of the top 20 oncology journals is given in Table 10.1, ranked by impact factor, which is defined as:

Table 10.1 The top 20 oncology journals of 2013, as ranked by impact factor

Rank	Journal	Impact factor
1	*Ca-A Cancer Journal for Clinicians*	162.5
2	*Nature Reviews Oncology*	37.912
3	*Cancer Cell*	27.238
4	*Lancet Oncology*	24.229
5	*Journal of Clinical Oncology*	18.038
6	*Cancer Discovery*	15.929
7	*Nature Reviews Clinical Oncology*	15.696
8	*Journal of the National Cancer Institute*	15.161
9	*Cancer Research*	9.284
10	*Drug Resistance Updates*	8.816
11	*Clinical Cancer Research*	8.193
12	*Biochimica et Biophysica Acta—Reviews on Cancer*	7.584
13	*Oncotarget*	6.63
14	*Annals of Oncology*	6.578
15	*Cancer and Metastasis Reviews*	6.449
16	*Advances in Cancer Research*	6.351
17	*Molecular Cancer Therapeutics*	6.107
18	*Breast Cancer Research*	5.88
19	*Journal of Thoracic Oncology*	5.8
20	*Journal of Mammary Gland Biology and Neoplasia*	5

The number of *citations* in a year (e.g. 2004) to articles published in the journal in the previous two years (i.e. 2002 and 2003) DIVIDED BY The number of *articles* published in the journal in those two years.

Editors therefore must attract relevant, high-quality research, which informs the work of others and is therefore cited by them, while maintaining a high rejection rate and tight control of the number of articles published each year. When Professor David Kerr began his tenure as Editor-in-Chief of *Annals of Oncology*, rejection rates were 50 %, but had risen to 85 % 8 years later, with a significant rise in impact factor (from 2 to 5.6). However, impact factor has its detractors as the ultimate ranking consideration because:

- Journal impact factors correlate poorly with actual citations of individual articles
- Authors use many criteria other than impact when submitting to journals
- Citations to "non-citable" items are erroneously included in the Web of Science database, which is used to calculate the denominator of the impact factor
- Self-citations are not corrected for
- Review articles are heavily cited and inflate the impact factor
- Long articles collect many citations and give high journal impact factors
- Short publication lag allows many short-term journal self-citations and gives a high journal impact factor
- The database has an English language bias
- The database is dominated by American publications
- Small research fields tend to lack journals with high impact
- Relations between fields (clinical vs. basic research, for example) strongly determine the journal impact factor

Nevertheless, it is a target for young researchers to aim for higher impact journals.

National or regional journals can be important for three reasons; as a repository for knowledge of most relevance to particular geographies; as a starting point for young researchers seeking to establish themselves; and, as a means of challenging English as the only language of science. The problem is that national journals often have difficulty in climbing the "impact factor league table" and are often deserted as the quality of research rises and there is pressure on individual scientists and clinicians to publish in international journals for promotion, etc.

Open Access Publishing

The kinds of publications that are accepted as contributions of knowledge or research vary greatly between fields; from print to the electronic format. A study suggests that researchers should not give great consideration to findings that are not frequently replicated. It has also been suggested that all published studies should be subjected to some measure for assessing validity or reliability to prevent the publication of unproven findings.

Business models are different in the electronic environment. Since the early 1990s, licensing of electronic resources, particularly journals, has been very common. A major trend, particularly with respect to scholarly journals, is open access. There are two main forms of open access: open access publishing, in which the articles or the whole journal is freely available from the time of publication, and self-archiving, where the author makes a copy of their own work freely available on the web.

While over a million scholarly articles are published every year in around 25,000 journals, only 20 % are freely accessible. In response to this, many Western governments have committed to expanding access to publicly funded research publications and data.

The most prevalent current approach in the scientific community is to publish results in subscription journals and pay-to-access websites. These channels of access can require considerable funding, however, just as they can generate huge revenue for publishing houses. Either way, free publicly accessible research is a commodity that can be hard to come by—not least the developing world.

The economic market of scientific publishing was described as complex in a report commissioned by the Wellcome Trust in 2003 [3]. There are currently two models of publishing used in the "first world" of scientific research. The first is a "subscriber-pays" model, the business model in which the journals are paid for by their individual readers and institutions by either a one-off fee or an annual subscription. These journals can be either in electronic format or traditional paper-based. The second model, "author pays," describes the situation in which the authors pay for the publication fee, which generally includes a submission and a publication element. It is not clear which of these models is most appropriate for publishing in the developing world. More acceptable would be that emerging results from less-industrialized nations' research could be published, or at least accessed, in a free or minimal-cost market. This could be a novel direction for existing journals and publishing houses and could result in the establishment of continent-specific platforms.

In addition to the cost models, publishers can be categorized into three distinct categories, as outlined in the Wellcome Trust report [3]. Commercial publishers understandably have the primary intent of capitalizing on any profit. University press-based houses prioritize publishing pieces of research excellence, with associated profit. Whereas not-for-profit institutions and so-called learned societies aim to publish results that further their specific areas of research interest. The question is: should there be the development of a fourth model specific to developing nations?

There are many clear advantages to open-access publishing, as outlined above. However, we need to proceed with caution in this developing sphere of publishing. The field of open access has grown exponentially over the past 10 years and is now a global industry, unfortunately often driven by large author subscriptions as opposed to the more traditional reader-paid approach.

This issue was highlighted by a piece of scientific journal investigation published in *Science* in 2013 [4]. The authors wrote a spoof paper, purporting to having identified novel anticancer properties of lichen. On closer inspection, the paper is littered with flaws, so basic that the authors state it should have been rejected by anyone with more than a high-school knowledge of chemistry. Rather than instant rejection, however, the paper was astonishingly accepted by half of the journals to which it was submitted, just over 150 in total. Perhaps more concerning was that the majority of these decisions occurred without peer review.

Several of the accepting journals were also misleading about their geographical location. For example, the *American Journal of Medical and Dental Sciences* is actually published in Pakistan. Such a misleading fact would surely not be tolerated in other modes of reporting, such as news journalism.

Furthermore, the editorial boards and, perhaps more pertinently, the financial dealings of such businesses are difficult to penetrate and lack clarity. Indeed, many of the accepting journals required significant up-front funds for publication—one journal requested a fee of $3100 to facilitate the publishing process. Significantly, the invoices for the publishing fees exposed a network of bank accounts, the majority of which were within developing nations.

Such obvious shortcomings need to be addressed if this format is to represent the mainstay of future result publication within the scientific community. The submission of a paper to a less-discerning journal is a temptation that junior researchers must resist, a difficult task in such a numbers-driven arena [5, 6].

Access to Results

It is essential for an efficient research community that scientists are able to access results at local, regional, and national levels. Following on from the example of the National Institute of Health Research (NIHR) Clinical Research Network (CRN)'s new platform, the Open Data Platform, the ultimate aim would be for basic results to be available freely and at real-time [7]. The necessity of this is many-fold; firstly, all participants of research would be able to identify what research is currently being undertaken. This would prevent duplication of results and lead to a more streamlined process, of paramount importance in resource-critical environments such as developing nations. To ensure clarity, the creation of a registry of current research activities, accessible to all, would be useful.

Secondly, we believe that the access to real-time results would permit research to occur in a more rapid and efficient manner—results could be accessed prior to publication, which would allow researchers to direct their projects or interpret results in a time-critical manner. But how far should the access to real-time results extend— should all individual results be available, including basic science or should the results be those that involve patient data only? A further consideration needs to be that only appropriate people—i.e., members of a specific research community, have access to the results. This is especially important if accessed results involve patient data; obviously all data would have to remain anonymous with no potentially identifiable features. One way to ensure that results are appropriately accessed would be to provide a simple yet secure login system whereby researchers obtain a unique username and secure password following verification of who they are. Administrators of the open-access platform would have to ensure not only that the platform is robust and could tolerate expected internet traffic, but that it is also a secure site.

There are obvious caveats to real-time data platforms that require further discussion—any intellectual property or ownership of results would still need to belong to the original authors; by not doing so we would risk that the most promising results remain "under the radar" until publication, which would undermine the collaborative nature of the research. Secondly, it would be important to highlight to any junior researchers that the results are available in a state prior to peer-reviewed publication. They would therefore require utilization of their analytical skills. There would also be significant pressure on the researchers to ensure that the results they are releasing are accurate—it is possible that groups would hold back results until they are confident of their accuracy, thus negating the real-time ideal.

Ultimately, the benefits of any scientific research are primarily derived from appropriate access to the results [3].

Application of Results

What is the point of clinical research if it does not influence medical practices? Research should not be a purely academic exercise; the ultimate aim is for research to direct medical management, so we deliver the most effective, efficient, and up-to-date treatment options to our patients. Furthermore, there is a responsibility that public investment in research has a demonstrable benefit to patient care, especially in the current economic climate, as resources become more limited and demands increase.

For excellence in clinical care, we need to train health professionals so that active uptake of the latest research findings into everyday practice is the accepted norm, moving away from the more traditional approach of passive diffusion of information and change to practice. There are several reasons why research findings may be slow to influence practice. These include obstructed access to information at the pertinent moment; individual and institutional barriers to change; and a lack of uniform medical practice within a professional body.

Health professionals constantly work under time pressure, confounded by increasingly distant targets and seemingly never-ending paperwork. As such, any relevant information needs to be easily accessible, up-to-date, and relevant. With today's technology, it should be possible for such information to be available at a click of a button. Automatic reminders on clinical systems could and should provide clinicians with the most up-to-date, research-driven guidelines. The only obstacle to this is the multitude of different clinical software programs that exist not only within national health systems but also internationally.

Implementation of Knowledge

Research results should influence all aspects of medicine—from an individual's medical management to influencing local, national, and international programs and policy making.

There are several steps, as follows, that should be followed to ensure that research findings are appropriately integrated (Adapted from Haines and Donald, 1998) [7].

1. Identify a gap between research findings and current medical practice
2. Precisely define the message to be delivered
3. Identify what needs to be modified in terms of current behavior
4. Recognize any potential barriers to behavior change
5. Determine interventions that will facilitate change—for example the development of clinical guidelines, or automated update reminders
6. Ultimately, through the use of clinical audits, identify whether the behavior change has a benefit to patient care

The characteristics of the message to be delivered are also important. It should be appropriate, generally applicable, up-to-date (with intrinsic mechanisms to update when necessary), valid and, importantly, clear, concise, and easy to digest. The message also needs a clearly defined audience.

Determining which results should influence change is often a far from straightforward decision. Not all published results should influence medical management, some are clearly not appropriate, and for the majority of others there needs to be clear prioritization. What determines prioritization is multifold; the quality of the research, the understanding of the subject to date, the relevance to current practice, financial implications and, ultimately, the ratio of potential costs to benefits.

Cost–benefit analysis determines whether the gain from treatment is significant enough to ameliorate the potential associated risks, both in terms of patient health and financial burden. Such cost-to-benefit analysis is often a hot topic in oncology. There are novel anticancer therapies that come to the market every year, extending life expectancy often by only months, but coming with significant financial cost. To help with decision making, policy makers often utilize tools to determine an overall figure of cost-effectiveness. This facilitates the establishment of a threshold, above which treatment is determined to be inefficient. Examples of such tools are numbers needed to treat (NNT) or quality-adjusted life years (QALYS), which have a fixed financial threshold. Both of these equations have recognized disadvantages; however, they remain staple tools in decision making [8, 9]. These calculations have to be made for individual interventions, as they are likely to differ in terms of overall benefits and risks to patients, and associated financial costs.

It is not always immediately obvious whether general research findings should be directly applied to a particular patient. Analysis of how research findings or new guidelines affect patient care is often based on average results across a sample population, therefore careful consideration should be made when making decisions for an individual patient. There are certain questions that need to be addressed:

- Is the calculated risk reduction likely to differ for this particular patient?
- Does this patient have any comorbidities that could influence any benefits or risks of the proposed management?
- Are there any social or cultural issues that may affect suitability?
- What does the patient want? This is a pertinent point as we move away from the traditional paternalistic doctor–patient relationship to the more equal relationship of today, with emphasis on concordance and shared decision making.

Ultimate Pathway from Research to Patient's Bedside

The schematic below (Fig. 10.1), adapted from Haynes and Haines [10], represents a simplified route from the benchside to the patient's bedside.

The majority of primary research is, as discussed, published in peer-reviewed journals. However, one of the main tasks for clinicians and policy makers alike is to determine the most clinically relevant findings from the wealth of published papers. One vehicle to overcome this task is delivered by the Cochrane Library, which accumulates, summarizes, and publishes the most salient points.

Developing Evidence-Based Clinical Policies

In addition to making the clinical decision for the individual patient, the evidence should be used to determine national and international guidelines. However, it is not only simply a case of choosing the new treatment option that has the greatest effect for the patient, but is also deeply influenced by financial constraints, available resources, and the disease itself. What is the population burden? What is the average patient demographic? What treatment options are currently available and how effective are they? These elements can obviously vary significantly from country to country, and especially between developed and developing countries. Whereas the ultimate pinnacle of policymaking would be a uniform guideline, which can be applied across continents. This is unlikely to be achievable due to different disease pathology, patient demographics, infrastructure, and available resources. It is certainly feasible that guidelines could exist for partner countries that share similar traits, for example, countries of sub-Saharan Africa. This, in theory, could streamline management with shared policy making, thus reducing administrative costs at the very least.

Application of Novel Treatment Options

The most robust clinical research is randomized control trials, which permit the unbiased study of treatment(s) on a specified group of patients, often stratified against certain demographics. By their very nature, the overall results published are

Primary research

↓

Accumulation of evidence

↓

Development of evidence based clinical policies

↓

Clinical decision -influenced by patient's demographics, disease profile, co-morbidities and wishes

Fig. 10.1 Pathway from benchside to patient's bedside

the average, and thus may be very different when applied to the patient in question [11]. The clinician must then try to approximate these results to their patient and make a recommendation. Most clinicians make this calculation based on intuition reinforced by years of practical clinical experience [12]. It would be more robust if this could be supplemented with (as opposed to replaced by) a decision-making tool. We envisage that within new guidelines there could be the provision of a decision-making algorithm that could allow the clinician to make some basic assumptions about their age, ethnicity, and comorbidities, etc. This certainly exists in a basic form, for example the latest guidelines for initiating antihypertensive therapy within the United Kingdom divides patient groups into age and ethnicity, and then recommends specific treatment options [9]. We propose extending such algorithms to include patient variables such as comorbidities and potentially extending them to include disease profiles, for example, tissue pathology.

Application of Research Findings in Developing Countries

The use of evidence-based guidelines is perhaps even more pertinent in developing countries as financial and healthcare resources are so limited, therefore necessitating the most efficient of all treatment options [13]. There are further challenges that policy makers and clinicians face in developing countries, for example, the populations often have a different spectrum of comorbidities, poor health awareness, difficult (sometimes impossible) access to healthcare, and different social and cultural beliefs.

In developing countries, where health finances can, in some situations, be limited to less than a £7 a day per capita [14], the pressures of the new guidelines being successful are significant. The consequences of this are that not only national healthcare budgets may be affected, but also any inefficient guidelines may directly worsen an individual's poverty state.

It has been asked whether it is possible to successfully manage cancer in low-income countries for a dollar a day [15], a figure within the reach of most developing countries. For significant, efficient, and beneficial medical care to be available at this sort of cost, it is most likely that it will have to occur in a more blanket approach, which would be further facilitated by a clear guideline. The Africa Oxford Cancer Foundation is planning a trial of tamoxifen in women with breast lumps clinically detectable at informal breast clinics [16]. These women cannot afford formal pathological diagnosis and the tamoxifen will be provided free of charge. It is hoped that the tumor burden could be reduced in up to 50 % of patients. If the initial results are promising and are made immediately and freely accessible to other clinician scientists, the hope would be that such policy could be extended to other countries with similar disease burdens, significantly reducing the timeline from results to policy development.

Developing nations often have a different health burden from their more industrialized neighbors. Most developing countries need to prioritize healthcare on the main illness that causes the majority of morbidity and mortality—commonly malaria, HIV, cancer, and overall child mortality. As the average life expectancy is comparatively young in developing nations, they have minimal need for guidance for illnesses that primarily affect older age, for example dementia. For country-specific guidance, and ultimately for independence, the aim would be for the developing countries to lead their own research programs. This would ensure that not only would guidelines be tailored to conditions that are the highest local medical burden, but that the clinical data reflect any local skewing in terms of the patient or disease profile.

Ultimately, up-to-date research has the ability to benefit all treatment, whether being applied in a developing or developed country. One important consideration is that the resources available to implement such treatment can vary between countries. Consideration regarding the extent of resources available needs to take place when writing local guidelines in developing countries. As physicians, we want what is best for our patients, especially when viable treatment options exist. In resource-deprived countries, policymakers and healthcare professionals need to ensure that limited budgets are spent most appropriately—a difficult task. Local and national policies need to be decided upon by a board of physicians, public health teams, and health economists. If the guidelines sufficiently influence local policy such that adjustments are needed to national budgets, this would also need government participation and agreement.

We are entering an exciting time for medical research and for the dissemination of results and development of guidelines in both developed and developing countries.

References

1. Decca Aitkenhead. Peter Higgs interview: 'I have this kind of underlying incompetence'. The Guardian Newspaper. http://www.theguardian.com/science/2013/dec/06/peter-higgs-interview-underlying-incompitence (2013). Accessed 10 June 2015.
2. Rennie D, Flanagin A, Smith R, Smith J. Fifth international congress on peer review and biomedical publication: call for research. JAMA. 2003;289:1438.
3. Wellcome Trust. Costs and business models in scientific research publishing. London: Wellcome Trust; 2004.
4. Hawkes N. BMJ news: Spoof research paper is accepted by 157 journals. BMJ. 2013; **347**: f5975.
5. Bohannon J. Who's afraid of peer review? Science. 2013;342:60–5.
6. National Institute of Health Research's Open Data Platform. The Open Data Platform. www.nationalarchives.gov.uk. Accessed 10 June 2015.
7. Haines A, Donald A. Making better use of research findings. BMJ. 1998;317:72.
8. Hutton JL. Number needed to treat and number needed to harm are not the best way to report. Br J Haematol. 2009;146(1):27–30.
9. Measuring effectiveness and cost effectiveness: the QALY. National Institute for Health and Clinical Excellence. https://www.nice.org.uk/proxy/?sourceurl=http:://www.nice.org.uk/newsroom/features/measuringeffectivenessandcostffectivenesstheqaly.jsp (2010). Accessed 10 June 2015.
10. Haynes B, Haines A. Barriers and bridges to evidence based clinical practice. BMJ. 1998;317:273.
11. Glasziou PP, Irwig LM. An evidence based approach to individualising treatment. BMJ. 1995;311:1356–9.

12. Lilford RJ, Pauker SG, Braunholtz DA, Chard J. Decision analysis and the implementation of research findings. BMJ. 1998;317:405.
13. Garnera P, Kaleb R, Dicksona R, Dansc T, Salinasd R. Implementing research findings in developing Countries. BMJ. 1998;317:531.
14. National Audit Office, Overseas Development Administration. Health and population overseas aid: report by the Comptroller and Auditor General. London: National Audit Office, 1995.
15. Kerr DJ, Midgley R. Can we treat cancer for a dollar a day? Guidelines for low-income countries. N Engl J Med. 2010;363:9.
16. Africa Oxford Cancer Foundation. www.Afrox.org. Accessed 10 June 2015.

Further Reading

Committee on Publication Ethics. http://publicationethics.org/
The EQUATOR Network. http://www.equator-network.org
Mayfield Handbook of Technical & Scientific Writing. http://www.mhhe.com/mayfieldpub/tsw/home.htm
International Committee of Medical Journal Editors. Uniform Requirements for Manuscripts Submitted to Biomedical Journals: Writing and Editing for Biomedical Publication. http://www.icmje.org/
Hypertension: Clinical management of primary hypertension in adults. NICE guidance, August 2011, 127.

Index

© Springer International Publishing Switzerland 2016
D.C. Stefan (ed.), *Cancer Research and Clinical Trials
in Developing Countries*, DOI 10.1007/978-3-319-18443-2

213

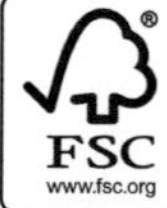

MIX
Papier aus verantwortungsvollen Quellen
Paper from responsible sources
FSC® C105338

If you have any concerns about our products,
you can contact us on
ProductSafety@springernature.com

In case Publisher is established outside the EU,
the EU authorized representative is:
Springer Nature Customer Service Center GmbH
Europaplatz 3, 69115 Heidelberg, Germany

Printed by Libri Plureos GmbH
in Hamburg, Germany